With support from the W.K. Kellogg Foundation, the National Academy of Sciences' Institute of Medicine sponsored a symposium to explore various alternatives for the provision of dental care under a national prepaid program. These papers, the result of that symposium, represent the ideas of an international panel of experts gathered by the Institute in cooperation with the Pan American Health Organization to examine worldwide approaches to dental care delivery programs. Since the United States appears to be on the verge of adopting a comprehensive unified national health program, these examples of various nations' approaches to solving the dental manpower program are most timely.

John I. Ingle is a graduate of Northwestern University Dental School, with further specialty training at the University of Michigan. The author of a leading dental text, Dr. Ingle spent twenty-four years in academic dentristry; sixteen years at the University of Washington and eight years as dean of the School of Dentistry at the University of Southern California.

Dr. Ingle presently serves as Senior Professional Associate at the Institute of Medicine. As a worldwide consultant, his interest in international dental care delivery methods is broad and long standing.

Patricia Blair, who holds degrees from Wellesley and Haverford colleges, has written numerous articles and monographs on the economic, social and political development of the Third World. Her most recent project involved work with the National Academy of Sciences on preparations for the United Nations Conference on Science and Technology for Development. Formerly editor of Development Digest, Ms. Blair is a member of the international Governing Council of the Society for International Development.

International
Dental Care
Delivery Systems

The Institute of Medicine
2101 Constitution Ave., N.W.
Washington, D.C. 20418
(202) 389-6958

The Institute of Medicine was chartered in 1970 by the National Academy of Sciences to enlist distinguished members of medical and other professions for the examination of policy matters pertaining to the health of the public. In this, the institute acts under both the academy's 1863 congressional charter responsibility to be an advisor to the federal government and its own initiative in identifying issues of medical care, research, and education.

The Pan American Health Organization
523 23rd Street, N.W.
Washington, D.C. 20037

The Pan American Health Organization (PAHO), first established in 1902 by eleven American republics as the Pan American Sanitary Bureau, is the world's oldest international health body. Since 1949, PAHO has served as the regional office for the Americas of the World Health Organization (WHO). Today, PAHO serves thirty nations of the Western Hemisphere. International headquarters are in Washington, D.C., with field activities administered through six zonal offices located in Caracas, Mexico City, Guatemala City, Lima, Brazilia, and Buenos Aires.

The PAHO dental health program serves to improve the practice of dentistry and the ability of countries and the profession to provide more preventive and curative services to the public.

International Dental Care Delivery Systems

Issues in Dental Health Policies

Edited by
John I. Ingle
Patricia Blair

*Proceedings of a Colloquium
sponsored by*

The Institute of Medicine
and
The Pan American Health Organization

Published for, and with The Support of, The
W.K. Kellogg Foundation, Battle Creek, Michigan

Ballinger Publishing Company • Cambridge, Massachusetts
A Subsidiary of J.B. Lippincott Company

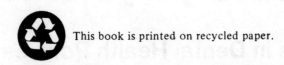
International Standard Book Number: 0−88410−529−6

Library of Congress Catalog Card Number: 78−13352

Printed in the United States of America

Library of Congress Cataloging in Publication Data

Main entry under title:

International dental care delivery systems.

At head of title: The Institute of Medicine and the Pan American Health Organization.
1. Dental care—Congresses. 2. Dental policy—Congresses.
I. Ingle, John Ide. II. Blair, Patricia. III. Institute of Medicine.
IV. Pan American Health Organization.
RK52.I57   362.1'9'76   78−13352
ISBN 0−88410−529−6

Contents

List of Tables

List of Figures

Foreword

The health professions are today facing public criticism on a number of fronts. Many Americans are questioning whether the professions should continue to have control of medical care and health services. It has been suggested, for example, that the dental profession has failed to publicly address the criticism of current dental health policy, to concede valid criticism, to offer sound rebuttals where criticism is demonstrably unwarranted, to admit where further inquiry and information are needed, to set up methods of gathering needed information, and to pursue these issues in every available public forum.

In early 1976, the W.K. Kellogg Foundation convened an Ad Hoc Advisory Committee on Dentistry that included representatives of dental education and dental practice and users of dental services. This group analyzed the situation as they perceived it very carefully and suggested future priorities for foundation consideration in programming with regard to dental health. Their overwhelming emphasis was on the need for more and better information by which the profession and the public could develop dental health policy. Among priorities selected for further development by the foundation staff were:

1. Development of professionally acceptable clinical standards and criteria for the assessment of dental care quality, including arrangements by which they can be practically and efficiently applied;

2. Support of demonstrations in community-based private practice setting utilizing expanded duty dental auxiliaries;
3. Support of efforts to develop better and more effective indicators of clinical need and effective demand for dental care as measurements for determining additional dental health manpower requirements;
4. Encouragement of efforts of the profession to outline the essential content of a model dental practice act; and
5. Encouragement of expanded efforts in the prepayment of dental care services, including experimentation with different modes of payments and delivery and with special attention to cost in relation to quality of care delivered.

The degree and ways in which the dental profession responds to such concerns will obviously greatly affect the future of the profession. It also will influence the dental health of Americans more than the simple exercise of current or new dental technique and technology. Moreover, the extent to which the dental profession will enjoy the continued confidence and support of the public—and avoid further intrusion and control by public bodies—will be a consequence of its response to these and related issues. Through grants in these five target areas, the Kellogg Foundation hopes to assist in the generation of needed information to provide a firmer basis for future dental health policy in the United States.

One of the earliest awards under this program was to the Institute of Medicine of the National Academy of Sciences', to undertake the consideration of various alternatives for the provision of dental care under a national prepaid program. In cooperation with the Pan American Health Organization, the institute began this work by convening an international panel of experts to examine worldwide approaches to dental care delivery programs.

As one of the few private philanthropic organizations focusing on problems of dental health, the W.K. Kellogg Foundation takes pride in having sponsored the international assembly and, through this publication, in broadening the potential reach and impact of the conference deliberations. This book is the first in a planned series of publications addressing "Issues in Dental Health Policy." This specific publication also should demonstrate, if a demonstration is needed, that nations have, among other things, much to learn from each other about dental care. Since its inception, the foundation has encouraged the intelligent application of knowledge to the problems of people. The overriding purpose of this new publication series is to further the attainment of that objective as it relates to the public's dental health. We hope you will find this volume a rich introduction to that theme.

Ben D. Barker, D.D.S.
Program Director
W.K. Kellogg Foundation

Preface

In preparing a proposal for an Institute of Medicine (IOM) study to deal with alternative methods for delivering dental care it was recognized that foreign models should be investigated as well as delivery systems employed in the United States.

Quite fortuitously, a meeting to discuss worldwide methods of delivering dental care was held in Havana, Cuba, in September 1976, sponsored by the Pan American Health Organization (PAHO). There was no doubt that a U.S. audience (and the IOM study) would benefit from such a program and the publication of the proceedings.

Hence an agreement was reached between the Institute of Medicine and PAHO to sponsor jointly an expanded version of the Havana meeting. A very generous grant from the W.K. Kellogg Foundation made that meeting and this publication possible. Held at the National Academy of Sciences in Washington, the discussions covered two full days—May 5 and 6, 1977.

In some measure the conference provided learning opportunities for all nations, developed and developing alike. In the jargon of the international development people, "technology transfer" should be the outcome. The United States, for example, could well make note of the community involvement in dental care delivery in such diverse cultures as Norway, Ecuador, and Mexico. Sweden's dramatic new preventive measures cry out for worldwide evaluation. The New Zealand expanded auxiliary legacy and Great Britain's efforts at cost containment demand widespread evaluation. Surely we can learn from the socialist nations as they learn from us. These reports are also filled with appropriate technology—homegrown solutions to complex dental materiel problems.

The good news throughout the world is that we are learning to take our "Mahomet to the mountain," to simplify our operation as we take our programs to the people—where they live, where they work. The bad news is that rampant edentulism appears to have grown out of our carefully nurtured garden of caring for our children. Motivation for continuing oral health must be built into every delivery system.

In anticipation of publishing these proceedings each speaker at the colloquium was required to prepare a manuscript. In addition the entire meeting was recorded including all audience participation. The proceedings were then edited for brevity and clarity and returned to each author for any corrections or additions. As editors, we have taken the prerogative to change the order of the presentations to allow for a better flow of subject matter. If national statistics were missing from the author's copy we supplied the information from a publication* of the Overseas Development Council (ODC) and have so indicated (ODC). In addition, unless so indicated, "DMF" refers to DMF *tooth* throughout. For the most part the illustrations are those shown by the speakers during their presentations.

I would like to acknowledge how grateful I am to the following people for their devoted assistance in making this colloquium and publication a success:

Dr. Ben Barker of the W.K. Kellogg Foundation
Patricia Blair, superb and exacting editor
Dr. George Gillespie, PAHO Dental Director
Frances Walton who typed and retyped the many manuscripts
Nydia Webb, my secretary
The talented illustrators in the NAS Printing and Publishing
    Office.

I must also extend my infinite gratitude to the speakers at this conference. Many traveled outrageous distances to appear in Washington.

I also wish to thank those who served as moderators:

Robert M. Ball, Chester W. Douglass, George M. Gillespie,
I. Lawrence Kerr, Alvin K. Morris, Anne Scitovsky, and
Jeanne C. Sinkford.

---

*The United States and World Development: Agenda 1977. New York, London: Praeger Publishing Co., 1977.

Finally, I must thank Dr. Harold Hillenbrand for his superb summary of the entire colloquium.

John I. Ingle, D.D.S.
Washington, D.C.
1977

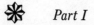 *Part I*

Introduction and Summary

Chapter 1

Greetings from the
Institute of Medicine

Dr. David A. Hamburg

One key feature of the Institute of Medicine is our strong interest in international health. We take a worldwide view of health. Thus, the Institute of Medicine is very pleased to cooperate with the Pan American Health Organization (PAHO) in this unusual conference. We are grateful to the PAHO leadership, Dr. John Ingle, and the W.K. Kellogg Foundation for making it possible. This conference reflects much imagination and much potentiality for future accomplishments.

All of us, from whatever country, profession, and walk of life, share rather precariously this highly interdependent planet that revolves through space and time. I have often thought that the major contribution of the space program was that marvelous photograph taken from the moon looking back at the earth—tiny earth. I never understood as vividly the interdependence of those of us who live on this small planet; that photograph captured and essence of it.

Now we must learn from each other in many ways, particularly in this century, when human activity has truly transformed the nature of life. Before the Industrial Revolution, our history was one of very slow social and technological change over the centuries. But today's human environment has been drastically transformed within the lifetimes of many of us. We are only beginning to learn the implications of this transformation for health and disease, for human relationships, for the view of life itself; and we are only beginning to understand the enormous problems, as well as the enormous benefits, that this transformation has brought.

Certainly, we must learn from each other how to improve health worldwide. We clearly cannot afford to be as parochial in this country as we sometimes have been in the past. We at the institute have been much impressed with what we can learn from developing countries. These countries are short of economic resources but long on human resources. In my activities at WHO, and during the years when I was conducting research in East Africa, I have been deeply impressed with the human ingenuity in poor countries—the diverse and remarkable ways in which imaginative people can respond to the challenge of very short resources to meet vital human needs. This in no way advocates that developing countries should remain economically poor, but their ingenuity in tackling health and other human service problems, even in the face of dire hardships, remains impressive.

We in the United States can also, of course, learn much from other industrialized countries about health care and social invention, because we are all groping our way. At the institute, we have had some very beneficial learning experiences. For example, in a study on polio immunization, we found that much of the truly critical data and informed judgments came from European countries. We have come to look to Canada for leadership in regard to prevention; this is symbolized in the now famous Lalonde Report and in the many activities undertaken in Canada to begin to implement the point of view—the New Perspective on Health—embodied in that report. In December I spent some time in Sweden, and last week I was in Israel. The scientific excellence and social ingenuity in those two small countries are really outstanding, even though their resources and the scale of their lives are much smaller than ours. With full appreciation of cultural diversity, there is much that nations can learn from each other pertinent to improving the health of their peoples. We at the Institute of Medicine are committed to fostering that kind of exchange based on mutual respect.

One important aspect of health, and one that is all too easily neglected, is dental health. You might suppose, from the "M" in our title, that the Institute of Medicine would not have such an interest, but we interpret medicine very broadly. Our charter, which goes back only seven years, requires us to emphasize factors pertinent to "the health of the public," and that is our interpretation of the "Medicine" in the title. Clearly, this means an important role for dental health. Because of our broad interpretation of what constitutes medicine in the modern era, our membership is drawn from all the health sciences and health professions; indeed, as provided in our charter, it goes beyond that in order to get multiple perspectives on any health issue we examine. Our council, our staff, and our study groups are also broadly composed in a national and international way and across the traditional disciplinary boundaries.

This conference provides the launching pad for a new major study supported by the W.K. Kellogg Foundation, which has a long and thoughtful interest in dental health. The program committee and the council of the Institute of Medicine have committed us to an analysis of key issues in national health insurance. We have decided that dental care for children is an important and manageable aspect of national health insurance that deserves our best analytical scrutiny. All of the major bills on national health insurance recently introduced into the United States Congress contain a clause that, in one way or another, calls for preventive and comprehensive dental care for children. The specified ages differ, but the general intent is clear. How to implement this excellent intent is not so clear at all. Except for the universal exclusion of orthodontics, the bills contain no definitions as to who will deliver this dental care, where it will be delivered, how it will be financed, or even what is meant by "preventive and comprehensive care." The institute believes that these and other facets of the problem should be explored as carefully as possible, starting now and using multiple perspectives to seek an overall public interest.

For a start, the Kellogg Foundation has agreed to fund an eighteen-month project on the delivery of dental care, as well as this conference on International Dental Care Delivery Systems. I am personally grateful to the executive officer of the Institute of Medicine, Karl Yordy, to John Ingle, and to Chester Douglass of the University of North Carolina, who is a former Robert Wood Johnson Fellow at the Institute of Medicine, for their key roles in formulating the study. To get it under way, we are fortunate to have been able to put together a distinguished committee. They are:

- Robert Ball, scholar in residence at the Institute of Medicine;
- Lois Cohen, special assistant to the director of the National Institute of Dental Research;
- Melvin Glasser, director of the Social Security Department of the United Auto Workers:
- Harold Hillenbrand, executive director emeritus of the American Dental Association;
- Lawrence Kerr, oral surgeon and trustee of the American Dental Association;
- Arden Miller, professor of maternal and child health, University of North Carolina;
- Alvin Morris, executive director of the Association for Academic Health Centers;
- Uwe Reinhardt, professor of economics, Princeton University;

- Dorothy Rice, director of the National Center for Health Statistics;
- Max Schoen, professor and chairman of preventive dentistry and public health at the University of California in Los Angeles;
- Anne Scitovsky, chief of the Health Economics Division of the Palo Alto Medical Research Foundation in California;
- Jean Sinkford, dean of the College of Dentistry at Howard University.

Some of the members of that committee are among the speakers at this conference and also—like the rest of us—among those who have come to learn from the experience of others.

ABOUT THE AUTHOR

Dr. David Hamburg became the third president of the Institute of Medicine in 1975. Prior to his return to Washington, Dr. Hamburg was Reed-Hodgson Professor of Human Biology in the Department of Psychiatry and Behavioral Sciences at the Stanford University School of Medicine. He also served for twelve years as chairman of the Department of Psychiatry at Stanford.

Dr. Hamburg has previously served in Washington with both the National Institute of Mental Health and the Walter Reed Army Institute of Research. He has also been a Sherman Fairchild Distinguished Scholar at the California Institute of Technology.

In 1947, Dr. Hamburg received his M.D. degree from Indiana University. His residencies in psychiatry were at Yale and at Michael Reese Hospital in Chicago.

His present address is: Institute of Medicine, 2101 Constitution Avenue, Washington, D.C. 20418

Chapter 2

Greetings from
the Pan American
Health Organization

Dr. José Luis García-Gutiérrez

This conference is the first collaborative effort in dental health between the Institute of Medicine and the Pan American Health Organization. And I believe it is the first occasion in which the delivery of dental services is discussed on such an extensive worldwide basis, bringing experience not only from the east and west but also from the north and south of the American countries.

The Pan American Health Organization has been extremely concerned with the need to develop new and effective methods to deliver health services. By the very nature of the region of the world for which we are responsible, this implies an urgent need to devise systems for a developing world in the Americas in which more than 40 percent of the population live in rural areas, 47 percent are without piped water supply, and, on average, 45 percent of the population are under twenty-one years of age. In response to this concern, the ministers of health of this region are actively searching for ways to meet the pressing health needs, with particular emphasis on rural and periurban populations where health resources are often limited or nonexistent.

In these past few months, we have conducted a series of meetings with multidisciplinary groups to assess regional health needs, not only in medical terms but also within their social and cultural contexts. Dental problems and actions are an integral part of this process. We are proud to note that this meeting today is an outgrowth of a workshop on dental health conducted by our dental section in September 1976 in Havana, Cuba, and are delighted to collaborate with the Institute of Medicine in this program. I should like to congratulate the staff of the Institute of Medicine for their initiative and hard work in making this meeting possible.

ABOUT THE AUTHOR

Dr. García-Gutiérrez is chief of the Division of Health Services with the Pan American Health Organization. Prior to coming to PAHO headquarters in Washington, Dr. García-Gutiérrez served as chief of PAHO Zone I in Caracas and as assistant chief of Zone II in Buenos Aires.

Dr. García-Gutiérrez received both his M.D. and Master's degrees in Public Health from the National Autonomous University of Mexico. His postgraduate residency was taken at Children's Hospital in Mexico City. Maternal and Child Health and Health Planning are his special areas of concern.

His present address is: 525 23rd Street, N.W., Washington, D.C. 20037

Chapter 3

Toward a Definition
of Questions

Dr. Julius B. Richmond

[*Dr. David Hamburg:* It is my pleasure to introduce Dr. Julius Richmond, a physician of great distinction, who has a long history of thoughtful interest in dental matters. He agreed some time ago to serve as chairman of the IOM Committee to Consider Alternative Dental Care Plans under a National Health Insurance Program. He was clearly the ideal chairman in the stature, vision and objectivity needed for the task. Dr. Richmond is well known as a leader in child health. With all the many notable years of his career at the University of Illinois, at the State University of New York, and at Harvard, and as a crucial member of the Institute of Medicine Council—one of the real builders of the Institute—Dr. Richmond has also distinguished himself in government service. He initiated the medical program in the Office of Economic Opportunity in its early days, directed it for a number of years, and has made exceptional contributions to the provision of health care for disadvantaged groups. Indeed, he has been an authentic pioneer in broadening the range of care available to those most in need. We were delighted when he agreed to serve as chairman of our committee, and my original plan was to introduce him as such.

However, there has been a change of plan, a change that is all to the good from the standpoint of the nation and the world, but a slight perturbation in our modest plans here at the Institute. I am happy and gratified to say that Dr. Richmond has just been designated as our nation's highest officer specifically and primarily concerned with health—the Assistant Secretary for Health in the Department of Health, Education, and Welfare. I offer my own personal congratulations, and I know we all join in wishing him every success and accomplishment in this important new position. He is a deeply respected leader in world health. He plans to stay with us through this meeting and through the first meeting of our committee in order to get us well launched, and then he will move on to his new position. It gives me great pleasure to introduce Dr. Julius Richmond.]

Dr. Julius Richmond: Thank you very much, Dr. Hamburg, for those very generous comments. It is a real pleasure to have an opportunity to attend this extremely important conference, which comes as the United States begins to reconsider the development of health services and, in particular, to consider building dental health services in a very integral way with general health services.

I might also lend a personal note to help explain my interest in this meeting and in chairing the Institute of Medicine (IOM) Committee on Alternative Dental Care Plans. I accepted with alacrity when I was asked to chair that committee, first, because I've always felt a genuine interest in oral health and its inclusion in general health and medicine, but second, and more specifically, because I have a deep sense of obligation to the dental profession. As a young medical student and teacher at Illinois, I came under the influence of Drs. Schour and Brodie and then collaborated with Dr. Sam Pruzansky, Dr. Milton Engle, and Dr. Maury Massler. They taught me, early on, the importance of oral health for the general health of children. They taught me, in addition, something I've valued very much—how to study growth and development. They also taught me the relationship of cranial-facial growth to general growth. That relationship and an understanding of it has had a great deal of meaning for me as I have proceeded in my various endeavors in child health and psychosocial development; indeed, my dental colleagues were quite influential in leading me to appreciate the importance of psychosocial development for the overall development of the child. I mention this for those who may be inclined to take a narrower view of dentistry, without realizing the importance of the relationship of psychosocial issues to oral health.

A comparative point of view is extremely important as we try to move toward more effective patterns of coping with the dental care problems we face in the United States. I am always reminded, when we talk about comparative views, of that old story of the internist and the biostatistician who were racing to their offices early one morning at the Clinical Center at the National Institutes of Health. They both managed to get into the elevator and, as it started to ascend, there was a moment of awkward silence. The internist, feeling uncomfortable, turned to the biostatistician and asked, "How's your wife this morning?" The latter thought for a moment and said, "Compared to what?" As we think about our problems, we need a comparative point of view. We need to look at models in other countries, the efforts other countries have made, many times with considerable success beyond our own in resolving some of their problems.

We face some very significant problems in this country in relation to dental care. To enumerate some of our problems just briefly, it is said that there are one billion unfilled cavities in the mouths of our population. Over fifty-six million teeth are extracted each year, and nearly twenty-three million people in our country—that is nearly 20 percent of our entire adult population are completely edentulous. These extractions, particularly among low income groups, are, we think, inordinately high. By age seventeen, the average adolescent will have lost 1.2 permanent teeth. By age forty-four, 10 percent of all the women in the United States are without teeth. In fact, the people in our country who go to dentists most often, the white female patients, end up the most edentulous; half of them are edentulous by age sixty-five and two-thirds by age seventy-five. Obviously, we need to take some steps to arrest this continuing march toward oral handicaps.

We are also aware that some segments of our population are underserved in relationship to dental care, and I'm thinking particularly of the low income population. When I was the first director of the Headstart program in the United States, we found that 75 percent of poor preschool children had never seen a dentist; indeed, half of the children in the United States under the age of fifteen have never been to a dentist. For those children who come into the Headstart program, we are generally able to provide dental services, but by and large, since most poor children are not in such programs, there remains a great deficit.

Dr. Harold Hillenbrand, the distinguished executive director emeritus of the American Dental Association, has made the following comment: "If we can arrange to bring up a generation of children in a state of good oral health, it will be relatively simple to maintain that condition as the child moves through adult life." This is what we should strive for.

In this conference, I think the important thing for us is to identify the critical questions and move toward developing recommendations that may provide some remediation for the problems we face. The matter of trying to find answers reminds me of a story about Gertrude Stein. As she lay on her deathbed, her followers gathered around. She was moaning, "What is the answer? What is the answer?" One of her followers, a bit bolder than the rest, said, "But, Gertrude, there is no answer." "Then," said Gertrude, "What is the question?" And I think that is what we must do—define the questions for which we need the answers.

ABOUT THE AUTHOR

Dr. Julius B. Richmond is the assistant secretary for health in the Department of Health Education and Welfare. He is also the surgeon general of the United States—U.S. Public Health Service.

At the time he made the remarks that make up Chapter 3, Dr. Richmond was director of the Judge Baker Guidance Center and psychiatrist in chief at the Children's Hospital in Boston. As such he was professor of child psychiatry and human development at Harvard University and professor of preventive and social medicine at Harvard Medical School.

Dr. Richmond was educated at the University of Illinois, receiving his Bachelor of Science degree in 1937 and Master of Science and M.D. degrees in 1939.

His present address is: Hubert Humphrey Building (Room 716—G), 200 Independence Avenue, S.W., Washington, D.C. 20201

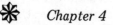

Chapter 4

What Can We Learn from Others?

Dr. Harold Hillenbrand

The United States is the only industrially developed country in the world without a coherent, identifiable national health program and has only now reached the stage of making a statement of intent— though frankly, I think we will have President Carter's balanced budget before we have a fully developed national health program. In the meantime, we can learn from the experience of other countries. That is one purpose of this Colloquium on International Dental Care Delivery Systems: to bring to our notice a vast amount of experience from other countries that have pioneered in this area. The Institute of Medicine's Committee to Consider Alternative Dental Care under a National Health Insurance Program is just beginning its work, and there is much to learn from the papers presented at this conference, no matter how much we have traveled or how much we have read about programs in other countries.

THE NEW ZEALAND LEGACY

When the dental history of our time is eventually written, I believe the New Zealand Dental Nurse Program will be considered one of the landmark developments in the practice of dentistry and dental public health. This program formalized and legalized the delegation of intra-oral professional operations to dental auxiliaries. Its degree of success has been debated, I would suggest, more than almost anything except motherhood.

Dr. R.K. Logan—who traveled 17,000 tiring, non-Concorde miles to get to this colloquium—concerns himself mainly with this dental nurse program, the dental profession's reaction to it, and its evolution over the past fifty years. Of particular interest is Dr. Logan's statement that New Zealand is now taking a hard look at the need for more dental health education in the program. I suspect that, in most of the countries of the world, there should be a new look at dental health education—whether it really does what we think it does and what the teachers say it does.

New Zealand has obviously pioneered in the development of a very effective method for delivering dental health services to children. It was the first country and the first profession to teach us that we do not need the anointed hands of the dentist to hold a cheek retractor. Furthermore, the New Zealand experience proves that we can develop an auxiliary program—and a very advanced one—that is acceptable to, and approved by, the dental profession of the country involved. As Dr. Logan points out, New Zealand dentists have no intention or desire to get away from the delegation of duties to auxiliaries. Although I recognize that this idea is highly controversial in some circles in the United States, I believe we ought to keep our eye on what has happened in New Zealand and on the rapid spread of the dental nurse concept, under appropriate controls and with appropriate variations, in many other countries.

Dr. Michael Lewis, of Canada, describes an innovative project that builds on the New Zealand experience. It was planned and initiated in Saskatchewan, presumably without the full cooperation of dentists and other establishment types. It is a skillfully designed project that does not give too much evidence of the compromises that must have been required to get it launched. The program seems to be off to a good start. Even though it began under something less than ideal conditions, careful planning is paying off, and experience is providing the basis for improvements and changes. The chief lesson for the dental profession, I think, is that it is better to meet a crisis in health care by consistent planning than by kangaroo jumps.

INNOVATIVE PROGRAMS
FROM THE AMERICAS

Dr. Gustavo Baz, of Mexico, tells about some of the difficulties of health planning in a country short of both manpower and financial resources. There are immense problems: the large rural population, which is hard to reach and needs much general and health education; a shortage of auxiliaries; perhaps a real shortage of dentists. But things have to begin somewhere, and Mexico is obviously trying hard to initiate a sound long-range dental health program. I suspect that we will soon begin to see real results in improved dental health in that country.

Dr. George Gillespie, of PAHO, discusses the Venezuelan program. I have seen that program several times, and it is very impressive. Its real heart is the active use of a university's resources. Personnel from the University of Zulia and its dental school have gone out into rural areas with an innovative program for using dental students and locally trained auxiliary personnel. They have also developed special equipment for use in these difficult areas. Most importantly, the teams do not go into a community without its full cooperation, so that auxiliary personnel can be trained at the local level to be competent enough to render adequate dental service. Dr. Gillespie pointed out that such a successful program deserves to be imitated. Ecuador has done just that, with encouraging government backing.

I know of no other country, except perhaps one in Africa, where an effort to train personnel locally in many population centers has been as effective as it appears to be in these two programs. I am pleased to see that something similar is also planned in Mexico.

Cuba is one of the rare examples of a dental health program developed almost exclusively from scratch, with problems of organization and a very serious shortage of dental personnel caused by the post-revolution exodus of more than 800 Cuban dentists. It would be interesting to know the schedule on which the Cuban program was developed because many questions are now being asked in the United States as to the schedule for a dental component in our own national health program. I am unable to make a good estimate myself, but Wilbur Cohen, one of the major architects of whatever national health system we have in this country, has predicted that the first real dental participation in the national health program would be more than thirty-two months after an initial bill was enacted.

As Dr. Silvino Miyares describes it, the Cuban approach seems to have been imaginative. It rests in large part on the development of dental auxiliary personnel, with the concomitant training of a larger work force of professional dentists. The emphasis is clearly on children's programs, and here again I note the use of the New Zealand type auxiliary nurse adapted for the special and local problems of Cuba. The ultimate objective is to provide free dental care for the entire adult Cuban population.

The Cuban program seems to me particularly well adapted for rural areas. In the United States, we have not yet given full attention to our rural area dental problems. Surely, in our own search for a national health program, we need to look more sharply at these questions.

SOME EUROPEAN EXAMPLES

One of my first assignments, when I became secretary of the American Dental Association in the mid-1940s, was to interview Aneurin Bevan, the minister of health and one of the principal architects of Britain's "cradle to grave" health scheme. Discussion of fluoridating communal water supplies was just getting under way at that time, and Mr. Bevan, who was well briefed indeed, asked me if it were correct that fluorides created fluorapatites on the surface of the tooth to act as a barrier to the caries process. I said, "How's that again?" and deflected the conversation to topics on which I was more knowledgeable. Mr. Bevan predicted that the United States would follow in the United Kingdom's path in health care—and sure enough, forty years later we are about to do just that. You may be sure that many in this country are studying and watching the British experience with a great deal of interest.

No matter how one evaluates the United Kingdom's National Health Service, one must admit that it was and is one of the greatest social experiments in health of our time. Dr. Michael Lennon gives a very impartial and objective view of the experience so far. He provides much information that many of us lack when appraising the program: how remuneration of dentists is really determined; the complexity of establishing fees; the difficulties encountered by government when there is inflation and dental demand is increasing. The crux of his message is that the National Health Service has learned how to deliver dental health care at relatively low cost to many people.

I do not think the British National Health Service will provide a precise pattern for the United States, except to indicate some areas into which we should not venture. For example, funding of the program must be examined more closely. It is frustrating for the profession, and certainly for Congress and the president, to find that cost estimates for a U.S. program are still horrendously divergent at this stage in our planning. I would guess that our estimates will also be far off the mark, as they were in Britain. Only a few months ago, an additional charge for dental care had to be placed on participants in the British National Health Service. How you correct bad estimates must be one of the most difficult aspects of conducting a national health program.

Dr. Jarmil Kostlán, of Czechoslovakia, offers a good view of a different type of program, with government heavily involved and a profession working without a cadre of trained dental auxiliaries. He describes how Czechoslovakia's program is developing under many of the usual handicaps. He notes the emphasis on dental care for children and the use of auxiliaries, though he seems less than ecstatic about the Czechoslovak use of medically, rather than dentally, trained nurses. It is evidently difficult and expensive to try to apply medical education and training immediately to dental practice. Dr. Kostlán indicates that the Czechoslovak dental health program has established a list of priorities, the first of which is to prevent tooth loss. The second priority is to provide fillings in preference to most other dental operations.

Dr. Kostlán is the only participant to introduce the subject of continuing education. In Czechoslovakia, he relates, every dentist must come back for an examination and, in effect, relicensure after three years. There are already signs that continuing education and relicensure will be part of a future national health program in the United States.

The system in Czechoslovakia works, or seems to work, without patient freedom to choose a dentist. In the United States, "free choice" has been a debating point from time immemorial. It would be interesting to examine, with the help of our sociological and behavioral colleagues, what the elimination of "free choice" really does to a system over a period of time. Hard information from patients in Czechoslovakia as to how they really feel about this would be more valuable than the usual guesswork found in our country.

Dr. Per Baerum, of Norway, offers a very common sense report on dental health delivery in his small and tidy country. What interests me is his statement that Norway is already detecting the directions in which its excellent and relatively young program ought to change. I think it exemplary that such flexibility can be built into a new program. A national health program needs constant examination and reexamination in the light of changing needs of the public, of professional resources, and of changing technology. Norwegian experience suggests that short-term evaluation, record keeping, and comparative data can provide the basis for evaluating and making changes. I would hope that the same type of information, retrieval, precautions, evaluations, and recommendations for change can be built into national health programs in the United States.

Dr. Jan Erik Ahlberg, formerly the secretary of the Swedish Dental Association and now the executive director of the Federation Dentaire Internationale, divides his presentation into three parts: a report on the Swedish dental program, a note on dentistry in the Netherlands, and a description of a preventive experience in plaque control. This presentation can only be exciting—nothing less—for those interested in the developing national health program in the

United States. Dr. Ahlberg's presentation is difficult to summarize, because it has many comparisons, lessons, and caveats for all interested in national health programs. It is highly quotable, but requires a close reading to get its full value and impact.

Sweden is a country at the other end of the spectrum from some of the countries reported on in these pages. It is highly developed, rich, and socially advanced and has a dental manpower pool that is very nearly more than adequate. It has a dentally oriented government, places its program emphasis on prevention and dental care for children, and manages to provide some benefits for adults. Dental care is provided through private practice and a national health service, thus frustrating the vocal prophets in the United States who equate any type of national health program with the elimination of private practice.

There are some surprises. Fluoridation is prohibited by law, there are 1.3 chairside assistants per dentist, the number of dental hygienists is very limited, and there are no expanded duty auxiliaries and no New Zealand type dental nurses. There are also some nonsurprises. Initial estimates of manpower needs and treatment targets turned out to be "gross misjudgments." A lack of epidemiologic data plagued the initial program stages with serious underestimates. As Dr. Ahlberg points out later in this volume, the initial effort to "create . . . a cheaper source of adult dental care open to all has failed." The "Swedish government . . . allowed the fee schedule to lag further and further behind real costs." The National Health Service has "not proved to be cost-effective." And again, "private practice caters at present to 80—85 percent of the dental care of adults and is expected to cover at least two-thirds of the adult population in the future."

Although the authority for the Swedish national health program stems from the central government, local councils bear heavy responsibility for its operation. Dr. Lennon, of the United Kingdom, and Dr. Baerum, of Norway, make the same point. I would think that this type of decentralization would have a great deal of appeal in the United States. Ours is a big country, and many of its citizens are a little wary of what goes on in Washington. They feel that decisions in health affairs like underwear, ought to be reasonably close to the people.

There is no question that the Swedish program should have the most serious study by planners in the United States. Its achievements and its deficiencies can provide a valuable model for this country.

Dr. Ahlberg comments briefly on dentistry in the Netherlands, where there is a dentist-population ratio of 1:3,500 and the national dental insurance scheme covers about 70 percent of the population.

There is a unique incentive program in the form of a "dental fitness card." This card is required for entry into the insurance program. If the patient is not "dentally fit," he receives some free treatment but must pay a part of the cost of restorative service. On completion of this work, the patient receives a dated "fitness card" and is notified to return in six months. Once the patient is fit, he receives free dental treatment and must pay only a part of the cost for fixed bridgework and full and partial dentures. If the patient does not return after the six month interval, he is classified as not "dentally fit" and must start the process all over again. Since a personal incentive for the patient is almost always the missing link in a national health program, the Netherlands experience is well worth noting.

TWO "CONTINENTAL" SYSTEMS

Dr. John Ingle tells us about dentistry in mainland China, with a rigid organization that provides very few options except at the governmental level. Almost everything is controlled by central regulations: the education and life of the dentist; fees, salaries, and practice locations.

I cannot conceive of transplanting the Chinese pattern to the United States any more than I can think of transplanting the U.S. pattern to China. There are differences—some of them real, some imagined, but all indicating that problems must be solved in the context of their own national systems and cultures. Nevertheless, the Chinese are doing some innovative things, such as combining Western medicine with the traditional practices of Oriental medicine. It would be interesting to send Dr. Ingle back some years from now to get another report, for we know very little of China's detailed program or how successful it will prove in the long run.

To my mind Dr. Max Schoen's chapter is the best review of dentistry in the United States that I have heard in a long time. There are some sharp conclusions, some good challenges, a lot of healthy skepticism, and some Schoenian recommendations that are bound to stir both imagination and controversy. Those from other countries will find Dr. Schoen's work a valuable, fact-filled reference source. Indeed, I discovered that I have been using some outmoded statistics, which will be replaced by those Dr. Schoen includes in his thoughtful and well-researched study.

NEW RESEARCH FINDINGS

Dr. Lois Cohen reports on an international cooperative study now under way in a cross-section of countries with a range of populations and a diversity of problems. She makes the point that health programs must be geared to the stage of development of the profession, to the realities of the culture, and to the form and resources of government. Sociological variables, I would think, are too often neglected in the development of national health programs.

On the basis of preliminary findings, Dr. Cohen also demythologizes some sacred and unsupported truisms relating to dental health programs. She notes, for example, that tooth loss is not necessarily related to disease patterns and that youth programs do not necessarily predict the success of adult programs. I find these statements stimulating because Dr. Cohen has the good grace to admit that she doesn't know something—implying, of course, that we don't either and that it would be a good idea for us to find the answers if we want to design an effective program.

Perhaps the most exciting single chapter in this collection is Dr. Ahlberg's report on the very significant work of Jan Lindhe and Per Axelsson, of Sweden, on a plaque control program for dental caries, gingivitis, and progressive periodontal disease. This demonstrates again the Swedish effort to make prevention a keystone of its national health program, thus decreasing the need for man hours and money presently devoted to reparative and restorative programs. If imitation in this area is flattery, we should flatter Sweden in developing our own health program.

Essentially, the Lindhe-Axelsson study reports on the effects of completely removing dental plaque by a combination of,"professional" tooth cleaning and tooth cleaning carried out at home. Both children and adults were evaluated in the longitudinal clinical trials. The results at three age levels, according to Dr. Ahlberg, were "startling." In the well-controlled study, over a period of three years, the test group children developed only forty-two new carious surfaces while the control group acquired 790 new lesions. Results in the other areas of the study were comparably startling. These studies are continuing and should have a major influence on the design of any national health program.

In summary, the studies from this colloquium reveal that we in the United States can learn much from other countries about effective delivery systems, about supplementing dental manpower with auxiliaries, and about daring to experiment with imaginative and innovative programs. They remind us that a major problem lies in meeting the needs of remote and rural areas and that there are no styrofoam models or cellophane-packed solutions available for every dental health problem. Most importantly, they remind us that there are not, and cannot be, any ideological variants in the dental profession's commitment to provide more and better care for all the peoples of the world.

There is, in these studies, substantial evidence that the dental profession must move in concert with many others in our society to improve the dental and total health of our nations. Inescapably— though these studies reveal a commendable eagerness to exchange ideas and to discuss both advances and disasters—the solutions to our problems must be found in the organizational, cultural, and social patterns of our individual times and countries. The systems for improving dental health in the world must be pluralistic.

Finally, I think one can conclude from this colloquium that the delivery of dental health care is not now, if it ever was, solely a problem for the dental profession. Real solutions must be found in the unselfish collaboration of dentists, the other health professions, the dental auxiliaries, social and behavioral scientists, epidemiologists, educators, statisticians, government and public health officials, consumers, and a whole host of others. There are enough problems to challenge and plague us all.

ABOUT THE AUTHOR

Dr. Harold Hillenbrand is executive director emeritus of the American Dental Association. His tenure as executive director of the ADA, and before that as editor of its journal, marked the zenith of the association to date.

Dr. Hillenbrand earned both his Bachelor of Science and D.D.S. degrees at Loyola University, Chicago. He is also the recipient of more honorary degrees and foreign decorations than any other member of the American dental profession.

His present address is: 211 East Chicago Avenue, Chicago, Illinois 60611.

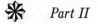 *Part II*

The New Zealand Legacy

Beginning only seven years after dental hygiene education was started in the United States, the New Zealand Dental Nurse Program is one of the oldest dental auxiliary programs in the world. Although the utilization of dental nurses was commended for consideration in the United States as early as 1934, it was not until 1948 that an abortive attempt was made in Massachusetts to train dental nurses.

Meanwhile, the movement spread worldwide, to Australia, Malaysia, and England in the New Cross auxiliaries, and finally to the province of Saskatchewan in Canada. Neighboring Manitoba has subsequently followed suit.

As we shall see in Part III, a number of Latin American nations have also picked up on the idea, each with its own variations.

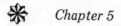

Chapter 5

Dental Care Delivery in New Zealand

Dr. Richard K. Logan

Area: 268,704 square kilometers
Population: 3,140,000
Per Capita Gross National Product: $4,310
Life Expectancy: seventy-two years

In New Zealand, dentistry has been provided for a long time as a collaborative effort between private dental practitioners and government agencies. Operating auxiliaries are well established. Private purchase of care by adults is supplemented by government payment for services to priority target groups, particularly young people and adults with special needs that cannot be met adequately through private practice. Fifty-four percent of the population is receiving the benefits of water fluoridation.

The distinctive feature of the New Zealand system of delivering dental care is its School Dental Service, which was instituted as early as 1921, under the leadership of the New Zealand Dental Association, to control the problem of caries, whose early onset and rapid progression has been the primary dental public health problem. The service provides preventive and restorative care for virtually all children up to the age of thirteen. It is staffed by specially trained dental auxiliaries—the school dental nurses who work within a closely coordinated, government-funded program.

It was only after caries control had achieved a measure of conservation of natural teeth for young people that periodontal disease was also recognized as a significant problem. Thus, the objectives of the School Dental Service today are more far-reaching than ever before.

OVERVIEW OF THE DENTAL CARE DELIVERY SYSTEM

While the School Dental Service constitutes a distinctive feature of the New Zealand system, it does not exist in isolation. Rather, it is one aspect of an integrated pattern of services, public and private, that have been evolving over a period of sixty years to meet the requirements of a total population. There is provision for orderly progression and referral from one service to another. Organizational relationships are well established, procedures are straightforward, and at least in theory, the total delivery system is efficient and effective.

Basic dental services are provided for the great majority of the population. They are the School Dental Service for children, the Social Security (Dental Benefits) Programme for adolescents, and private dental practitioners for adults. In addition, there are some special services for people of all ages who cannot make use of the basic services.

The School Dental Service for Children

Personnel of the New Zealand School Dental Service are distributed throughout the country to cover all schools, and every child has ready access to dental care from two and one-half to thirteen years of age. Apart from some specialist services, including orthodontics, the central government meets the total cost.

All primary and intermediate schools built for 450 or more pupils have small permanent field clinics that are either free standing or attached to the main school buildings. They are designed to accommodate two school dental nurses and are usually equipped with some fixed installations and some portable equipment. Schools for 250–400 pupils have smaller clinics, designed for part-time use by a single nurse. Altogether, there are 1,373 of these clinics to serve the children from the surrounding areas. There are also mobile clinics, but we have found it more economical to work from static clinics, even if we have to provide the nurse with transport.

Parental consent is mandatory for school children, who usually come directly from the classroom for examination or treatment. Preschoolers are brought to the clinics by their parents on regularly scheduled appointments. While the service is not compulsory, the utilization rate is very high—reaching 98 percent of primary and intermediate school children and 64 percent of preschoolers, for a total coverage of 622,000 and an average cost of $16.92 per child per year, not including staff training costs.

In fluoridated areas, dental nurses provide routine care at six month intervals for about 650 children; in nonfluoridated areas, for 450−500 children. The routine care offered is:

- Oral examination;
- Oral prophylaxis;
- Topical fluoride application and recommendation of dietary fluoride supplements where appropriate;
- Removal of incipient caries and caries-susceptible areas;
- Cavity preparation and placement of silver amalgam and silicate cement restorations in deciduous and permanent teeth;
- Polishing of all restorations;
- Administration of local anesthetics by infiltration and mandibular nerve block techniques;
- Pulp capping;
- Extraction of deciduous teeth;
- Individual patient counseling on toothbrushing techniques and oral hygiene;
- Classroom dental health education;
- Parent-teacher health education for influencing dietary habits and health practices in the home; and
- Referral of patients as required.

For many years, school dental nurses extracted permanent teeth, but when the need for this operation declined to a level of 0.3 permanent tooth extractions per nurse per year, teaching of the technique was discontinued. Radiographs are not taken by the nurses. Instead, children are referred to private practice for conditions requiring experienced radiographic diagnosis and for permanent tooth extractions.

Social Security (Dental Benefits) for Adolescents

For the adolescent population up to age sixteen or, if they remain dependent on their parents, eighteen, oral health care has been available as a Social Security Health Benefit since 1947. The program can be regarded as compulsory insurance in that it is funded by government out of general tax revenues. Service is provided by private dentists, in their own offices, under contract to the minister of health. In practice, more than 95 percent of general practitioners are contracting dentists, and about 85 percent of the target population is receiving care under this program at a cost per child of $25.40 a year.

The adolescent is enrolled at age thirteen with a contracting dentist of his parents' choice, but the dentist is free to accept or reject him, and enrollment can be terminated or transfer arranged at any time on request from either party. Each enrollment is recorded by the Department of Health, which pays the contracting dentist according to a schedule of fees negotiated with the New Zealand Dental Association. This method of payment has been criticized by both private and public dentists on the ground that it orients the program toward treatment rather than disease prevention and health promotion, but suggested alternatives have failed to gain acceptance.

The scope of treatment provided in the adolescent program is more comprehensive than that in the school program. It includes restorations in a wider range of materials and restorations for extensive tooth destruction from injury or other cause. Younger school children can be transferred to the program for adolescents if they need more complicated treatment. Again, some specialist services, including orthodontics, are excluded. Expenditures in 1975 were as follows:

Diagnostic and prophylactic services	35.5 percent
Routine restorations	58.0 percent
Periodontal and surgical treatment and nonroutine restorative services	6.5 percent

Private Dental Practitioners for Adults

The majority of adults purchase dental care on a direct fee for service basis from dentists in private practice. The rate of utilization has not been measured in precise terms, but surveys have indicated quite clearly that, for routine health maintenance, utilization is well below the levels achieved by the services for children and adolescents.

Supplementary Service for Special Groups

The central government pays for services to special groups that— for medical, psychological, social, or financial reasons—cannot make full use of the basic services. Members of the armed forces, prisoners, social welfare beneficiaries, and accident victims receive dental care in this way. Major hospitals have both in- and outpatient dental departments staffed by dentists and supporting personnel, and plans are being made for including dental services in multipurpose community health centers and polyclinics.

DENTAL MANPOWER

Dentists

The graduate dentist is the key person in dental care delivery. He is involved in planning and evaluating programs and in training and supervising auxiliary personnel, as well as in providing personal dental services through private practice and hospitals. Dentists are distributed reasonably satisfactorily through the population at a ratio of 1:2,880, or 1:2,310 if the school children treated by dental nurses are excluded.

There were 1,090 active dentists in New Zealand in 1976. About 86 percent of them were engaged in general or specialist private practice, primarily on their own. Group practices involving two or more dentists represented about 30 percent of all practices. Other dentists are employed full or part time in an institutional capacity—in public health administration, dental research, university teaching, training of auxiliary personnel, or as salaried dentists in the armed forces, hospitals, and state institutions and public health services.

All dentists are university graduates who have taken a five year course leading to the Bachelor of Dental Surgery. Both masters and doctorate degrees are offered in New Zealand (at Dunedin), as well as graduate study courses leading to the diploma in Dental Public Health. Since these courses are basically similar in content and standards to those in Australia, graduating degrees from both countries are recognized as a basis for certification to practice, and there is a free flow of dentists from country to country.

Dentists rank with professionals in medicine and law, high on the scale of occupational class incomes. Average net income is about $19,000—20,000. Only 2.7 percent of registered dentists in 1975 were women, but this situation will change rapidly. About 30 percent of recruits to dentistry today are women.

School Dental Nurses

There are currently 1,300 school dental nurses engaged in field service to care for a School Dental Service enrollment of 622,000 children. In addition, forty are engaged in tutoring and twenty in program management. They are government employees with salaries similar to those of teachers, nurses, and other paramedical groups. An experienced school dental nurse, after about five years, earns around $8,000. School dental nurses work under remote supervision of district dentists and dental nurse supervisors. The dental officers are primarily concerned with continuing training and quality control of clinical work. As dental nurse supervisors, they visit the clinics periodically to advise on clinic maintenance, work organization, and recording procedures.

Dental nurses undergo an intensive two year course with heavy emphasis on clinical experience. There are three schools for dental nurses—at Auckland, Wellington, and Christchurch—set up by the

Department of Public Health and run in association with large children's dental clinics. The schools are headed by principals, who are dentists, and staffed by graduate dental officers with training and experience in teaching methods. In addition, there are "tutor sisters," who are experienced dental nurses. The staff to student ratio is about one teacher to eight students. On completion of the two academic years of study and training, students are examined by boards of examiners that include practicing dentists.

New Zealand is today able to train more dental nurses than it needs, since the three schools have a capacity to graduate 220 a year, but only half that number are required annually. In 1977, student intake was reduced to 120. (Between 1973 and 1977, Australian trainees took up the slack capacity; under an agreement with the Australian government, about 100 of their dental therapists were trained.)

In part, this excess capacity is the result of an increase in the average career life of the New Zealand dental nurse. Before 1974, the average career life was about six or seven years. For some reason—perhaps having to do with smaller modern families, perhaps with job satisfaction—this average has increased to about ten years and is still going up. Some dental nurses have been encouraged to become dentists, but few have done so. So far, only one has graduated.

Other Auxiliary Personnel

Nonoperating dental auxiliaries, virtually all of them women, include chairside assistants (1,300, or about 1.3 per dentist), secretary-receptionists (500, some of whom are trained), and dental technicians (350, about one per three dentists). In addition, there are six active dental hygienists working in the armed services as part of defense dental teams. Hygienists receive seventeen weeks of training beyond that for regular chairside assistants; the latter usually start as medical orderlies or sickbay attendants, receive some formal training and experience, and move on to some aspect of medical or dental stores administration before becoming dental chairside assistants.

EVALUATION FROM THE 1930s
TO THE 1970s

The New Zealand school dental program was instituted as a trial project in 1921, long before dentistry developed an index for measuring, in quantitative terms, the distribution and severity of dental diseases in a community. It arose out of an intuitive assessment of the situation that existed in New Zealand in the first twenty years of this century—high caries prevalence, advanced destruction of teeth in both deciduous and early permanent dentitions, shortage of qualified dental manpower, and neglect of the need for dental care in early childhood.

Although it was obvious at the time that the most pressing demand would be for treatment to relieve pain and to eliminate gross oral sepsis, disease prevention and positive health promotion were to be characteristic features of the new program from the start. Today, we think of prevention in terms of specific techniques, but the early proponents of the program were thinking in more generic terms. The long-term aim was to promote positive health for the nation by giving priority to the needs of the young, by placing emphasis on providing incremental care for early caries rather than on providing crisis dentistry, and by locating the program in the learning environment of the schools where health education could be expected to flourish.

Between 1935 and 1939, public health administrators made a series of important further decisions based on their impressions of the successes and failures of the trial project. Some of these decisions were not implemented until after World War II, but they had far-reaching implications for the subsequent development of dentistry in New Zealand. These decisions were:

1. To make the school service permanent and to expand it to cover the total primary school population;
2. To extend the service to include preschoolers;
3. To develop a research component to include both epidemiological and operational management research;
4. To develop a dental health educational component by appointing a full-time dental officer and a group of dental nurses to direct and coordinate health education activities; and
5. To extend the advantages of routine surveillance and care to adolescents—which led to the introduction in 1947 of Social Security (Dental Benefits).

In the earliest years, there had been general optimism that the rampant caries affecting the total population could be dramatically reduced within a few years. We know now that that confidence was misplaced, but a series of evaluation exercises has produced evidence of steady progress toward the long-term goal.

One early objective was to increase target population coverage as quickly as resources would allow. Progress was rapid in the first few years, but it slowed during the economic Depression of the early 1930s and during the Second World War. A marked birthrate increase in the immediate postwar years was a further obstacle to progress. From the midfifties onward, however, the service expanded steadily until complete coverage was achieved (see Figure 5–1).

Another important objective in the early days was to reduce the tooth mortality rate. When the first group of trained school dental nurses entered field service in 1923, they extracted nearly as many teeth as they restored—78.6 extractions for every 100 restorations. Ten years later, the ratio had declined to 17.4 extractions per 100 restorations. Today, it is as low as 2.3 extractions per 100 restorations, and this figure includes some deciduous teeth due for exfoliation. As target population coverage increased, the need for extraction decreased. By 1970, the annual extraction rate was less than twenty teeth—nearly all of them deciduous—per 100 patients (see Figure 5–2).

From its inception, the School Dental Service adopted standard terminology and methods for reporting dental conditions and recording dental operations. The statistics were intended primarily for project management purposes, but they did provide a quantitative basis for initial evaluations.

The 1947 Survey of Child Dental Health
The first national survey of dental health of 22,000 children six to seventeen years old was undertaken in 1947.[1] This survey showed quite clearly that caries prevalence was still very high, even though the school service had achieved some success in limiting the more harmful effects of the disease. Comparison with similar surveys carried out in the United States at about the same time revealed several points: caries prevalence was substantially higher in New Zealand; the number of teeth extracted was lower; and the amount of restorative work performed was higher than in the United States, but some caries remained untreated. Significant decisions resulting from this survey were:

1. To establish a pilot fluoridation project, which led to a greater coverage of the population; and
2. To expand the teaching program in order to increase the school dental nurse to child population ratio.

The Beck Survey of Fifteen to Twenty-one Year Olds, 1963
By 1960, the programs for children and adolescents were well established. The time had arrived to study a population group that had been exposed to both programs. In 1963, Beck[2] carried out a

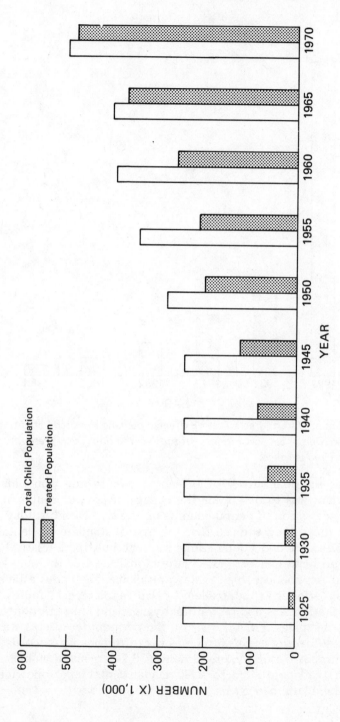

Figure 5–1. Proportion of Total School Population Enrolled in School Dental Service—Forty-five Years Experience. *(From a meager beginning in 1925, virtually every child is now involved. Fifty percent utilization was not reached until after World War II.)*

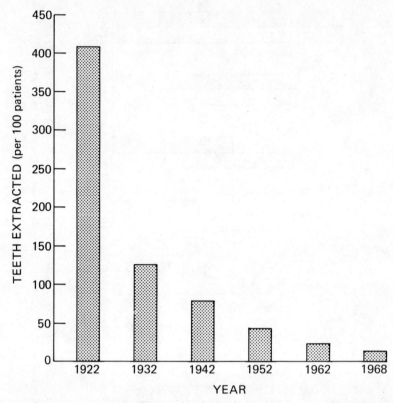

Figure 5-2. Number of Children's Teeth Extracted per One Hundred Patients Treated in School Dental Service. *(Permanent tooth extraction rate is presently only 0.0018 per child enrolled.)*

comprehensive national survey of fifteen to twenty-one year olds. The primary aim was to determine the change, if any, in dental fitness following cessation of dental benefits on the sixteenth birthday.

Results of the survey showed that the overall standard of dental health of adolescents and young adults was high but that a relatively minor caries problem existed, particularly in males. While the sample examined had experienced high caries prevalence, the caries attack rate had been effectively controlled by late adolescence. Indexes showed that the females had better oral hygiene and less periodontal disease than the males. For both sexes, the periodontal disease was mild and of a low order of prevalence. A sex difference was recorded in dental treatment history: more females (76.7 percent) than males (66.7 percent) had continued to seek regular dental care following cessation of the dental benefit.

One decision that arose from this study was to extend the dental benefits program to cover those adolescents up to age eighteen who remained dependent on their parents.

The International Collaborative Study
of Dental Manpower Systems

The next major study was the International Collaborative Study of Dental Manpower Systems, organized and directed by the World Health Organization and financed by the U.S. Public Health Service in the early 1970s. This was the first major attempt at an international comparison of dental systems, and New Zealand, represented by the Canterbury region, was one of the five collaborating countries.[3] Analysis of the vast amount of information collected in this survey is a mammoth task, which is continuing. This chapter will highlight only the preliminary results that are relevant to New Zealand.

The mean number of decayed, missing, and filled (DMF) teeth in thirteen and fourteen year old children in Canterbury was 10.7, the second highest of the five international regions selected (see p. 205). On this basis, Canterbury does not measure up very well, but if the raw DMF score of Canterbury could be adjusted—and there are valid grounds for adjustment—the figure would not be particularly distressing. Indeed, one could say that the New Zealand area scored as well as any other site sampled. For the simple fact is that, in the New Zealand sample, all but 0.6 caries had already been diagnosed and treated. The surveyors could do no more than count the number of filled teeth, since few remained decayed or were missing.

Accepting that caries is still a problem for thirteen and fourteen year old students—though reductions have been achieved in recent years—the data show that the problem has been brought under control without tooth loss. Ninety-four percent of the New Zealand DMF score represents filled teeth, with only 6.0 percent representing incremental caries, and less than 0.01 percent representing teeth missing because of caries. Using "quality of restorative dentistry" and "treatment required" as criteria, the data showed very few teeth with defective restorations; virtually no requirement for pulp treatments; no requirement for extractions because of caries; and gingivitis prevalence of a low order.

To summarize, at thirteen to fourteen years of age:

1. Caries had been treated,
2. Restorations were sound,
3. Tooth loss had not occurred, and
4. There was no periodontal disease problem.

When we look internationally at the total DMF scores for the thirty-five to forty-four year old groups, however, we find a very different picture.[4] Untreated caries account for smaller proportions of the total DMF scores than in the student samples, with the lowest treatment requirement for caries being in Canterbury. But the outstanding feature is the massive difference in the M(missing) component and the variability of the differences from nation to nation. In Canterbury, the M component (14.66) accounts for more than 50 percent of the total 22.0 adult score, with a higher rate of edentulism in females (40 percent) than males (30 percent). As might be expected, high percentages of the adult populations have either full or partial dentures (see Table 5-1). Although Canterbury shows the lowest incidence of periodontal disease of the five sites (see p. 208), it is nevertheless in the category defined by Russell as showing evidence of early destructive periodontal disease.

In sum, the dental health of Canterbury thirty-five to forty-four year olds, as revealed by the WHO survey, shows the following characteristics:

1. Relatively low prevalence of periodontal disease;
2. High caries experience;
3. Radical treatment, commonly extractions and dentures, rather than conservative care, with a high prevalence of full denture wearers; and
4. Low treatment needs apart from prosthetic replacements.

It is appropriate to remember that the Canterbury adults who were between thirty-five and forty-four in 1973 were born in 1929–1938

Table 5-1. **Disappointing High Percentage of New Zealand (Canterbury) Adults, Thirty-five to Forty-four Years of Age, Who Wore Some Form of Denture in 1973.** *(These patients were born in 1929–1938, when fewer than one-third of nation's children were treated by school dental nurses.)*

	Full	Full or Partial
Sydney	12.8	47
Trondelag	5.8	27
Canterbury	35.6	55
Hannover	2.0	23
Yamanashi	0	14

Source: World Health Organization—Division of Dentistry/International Collaborative Study of Dental Manpower.

and reached adolescence before the New Zealand program had been well developed. They did not receive the same dental care that is available to young people today. Thus, the WHO survey cannot be regarded as an objective evaluation of New Zealand's dental services as they are developed today.

The Cutress Survey of Adult Dental Health, 1976

Preliminary reports on dental aspects of the WHO study prompted organized dentistry in New Zealand to undertake its own comprehensive survey of adult dental health under the direction of T. W. Cutress. Collection of dental and sociological data was completed in 1976, with active participation of all dental organizations in New Zealand, including the dental unit of the Medical Research Council; the dental division of the Department of Health; the University of Otago Dental School; the University of Canterbury Department of Sociology; the New Zealand Dental Association; and the Defence Dental Services.

Analysis of the dental data has commenced, but the sociological data have not yet been examined. In an interim report,[5] Cutress showed that while caries prevalence was still high in late adolescence and early adulthood (fifteen to nineteen years) in 1976, a substantial reduction—from 16.7 to 13.4 DMF teeth—has occurred since Beck's 1963 survey. The mean number of missing teeth was as low as 0.3, and the number of teeth requiring extraction was very low, at 0.05. Edentulism appeared at a rate of 2 per 1,000, but the edentulous 0.2 percent came from the ranks of the 15 percent of adolescents who had ignored the opportunity to enroll for dental benefits.

Analysis of the dental data relating to fifteen to nineteen year olds confirmed the impression, widely held by New Zealand dentists, that government-funded services for children and adolescents had brought caries under control, with a substantial reduction in prevalence rates and without tooth loss. It confirmed also that the dental health of young people entering adult life in the 1970s is better than ever before in the history of New Zealand.

Analysis of dental data relating to the total adult population suggests, however, that the age level eighteen to nineteen years is a turning point in the dental lives of young New Zealanders. At eighteen, they pass beyond the tender care of the public health programs to encounter the grim realities of adult life—which include private purchase of dental care.

During the years twenty to twenty-four, tooth loss commences. In the years twenty-five to thirty, the rate of tooth loss increases. After sixty-five years of age, the mean number of missing teeth is twenty-five, and 73 percent of the population is edentulous. In the sample surveyed, the disease prevalence pattern does not, by itself, account for the progressive tooth loss that has occurred. According to the diagnostic criteria applied in the survey, the numbers of teeth requiring restorative treatment and of teeth requiring extraction were not particularly high at any age level.

Why, then, does this pattern persist? It is always said that there are two barriers to dental treatment—cost and pain. Pain does not seem to be a big factor in New Zealand. But there are other factors—the time spent in the dentist's waiting room, the inconvenience, the discomfort, the travel costs, and time spent in travel, among others. New Zealand has had a health education program going for a long time. Many methods have been tried, some with more success than others. The country has now entered an era where all the emphasis is on prevention and should, in the near future, expect to see a considerable drop in the need for restorative care. New Zealand has set an objective for 1977 to reduce the need for restorations in children by 10 percent, and it appears that this can be achieved. The nation is diversifying the program to meet the needs of local communities according to disease patterns. Beyond that, perhaps the dental professionals will have to turn to the sociologists and other behavioral scientists for an explanation of the interplay that has occurred between the providers and the consumers of dental services in New Zealand.

To sum up, an integrated pattern of dental services has been developing in New Zealand over a period of sixty years to meet the needs of a total population. Periodic evaluations have given rise to a series of modifications. In the past, evaluations have been planned, implemented, analyzed, and interpreted by dentists. Recent large-scale evaluation exercises have incorporated up to date dental epidemiological and sociological techniques. The behavioral scientists will be called upon in planning modifications for the future.

NOTES

1. R.E.T. Hewat, Field Studies on Dental Caries in New Zealand, *N.Z. Dental Journal* 44 (July 1948): 163–91.

2. D.J. Beck, *Dental Health Status of the New Zealand Population in Late Adolescence and Young Adulthood*, Special Report 29 (Wellington, New Zealand, R.E. Owen, Government Printer, 1968).

3. P.B.V. Hunter and P.B. Davis, Oral Health Care for Canterbury, New Zealand, 13–14 Year Old Students, *International Dental Journal* 26 (1976): 334–39.

4. E.D. Barmes, A Progress Report on Adult Data Analysis in the WHO/ USPHS International Collaborative Study (Presented at F.D.I. Congress, Athens, 1976); and P.B.V. Hunter and P.B. Davis, Unpublished Report.

5. T.W. Cutress, Unpublished Report.

ABOUT THE AUTHOR

Dr. Richard Logan is director of the Division of Dental Health in the Department of Health, New Zealand. Prior to assuming these national responsibilities, he was principal dental officer for Auckland, New Zealand.

Dr. Logan received his B.D.S. degree at the University of New Zealand and a Doctor of Public Health degree at the University of Sydney, Australia. As a demonstration of the respect between the island nations, Dr. Logan has been made a fellow of the Royal Australian College of Dental Surgeons.

His present address is: Department of Health, P.O. Box 5013, Wellington, New Zealand.

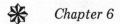 *Chapter 6*

Notes on Dental Care Delivery
in Australia

Dr. Richard K. Logan

Area: 7,686,850 square kilometers
Population: 13,500,000
Per Capita Gross National Product: $5,330 (1974)
Life Expectancy: seventy-two years

For the great majority of Australians, comprehensive dental services are offered only through private practice, on a direct fee for service basis. Government involvement has been minor, and experience in the use of operating auxiliaries is limited, although the scattered rural population receive some dental services through their state governments. State-supported "Outback" dental services, using railway rolling stock and aircraft, have been operating in New South Wales and Queensland for a very long time. The railway carriage, converted for use as a clinic, is shunted onto a small station siding where it remains until the people of the area have received the care they need. Like New Zealanders, Australians have a long history of high caries prevalence, high sucrose diets, and low fluoride water supplies.

SCHOOL DENTAL SERVICE

Today, government involvement in the delivery of dental care is increasing. After nearly fifty years, Australia is following the lead set by New Zealand in developing an operating auxiliary service for school children. The state of Tasmania started a small training program for dental auxiliaries in 1966, followed in 1967 by the state of South Australia. In 1973, an Australiawide school dental scheme was initiated through commonwealth-state cooperation, the main objective of which is to develop, within each state and territory, a comprehensive school dental service offering free dental care to all children under the age of fifteen, with emphasis on preventive care. Currently, there are 334 school dental clinics. Dental services for young people are still in an early stage of development, however.

Such school dental clinics as have been built reflect a somewhat different philosophy than those in New Zealand. Clinics are on a larger scale and often include operating facilities for a dentist who is assigned clinical, teaching, and supervisory functions in a cluster of clinics. In contrast to New Zealand, Australian dental nurses are trained to work with assistants. There are ninety-three mobile school dental clinics to help reach Australia's scattered population.

PRIVATE AND SALARIED PRACTICE

Other salaried dental services, mostly free of direct patient cost, are provided by the government for armed services, hospital inpatients, inmates of institutions, pensioners, and low income earners. Prepaid dental schemes cover a small proportion of the population, though the experience of a corporation formed for this type of service in 1974, under the sponsorship of the Australian Dental Association, appears to indicate that there is no great demand for this type of program.

DENTAL MANPOWER

Dentists

There are 5,006 active dentists in Australia, for a dentist to population ratio of 1:2,697. However, there are many areas where isolated communities do not have convenient access to dental services. The problem arises from the vastness of the country and the small, scattered nature of the population outside the large cities and towns. Seventy-two percent of Australian dentists are in general or specialist private practice, with perhaps a third in group practice and 11 percent employed by other private practitioners.

Auxiliaries

Dental auxiliaries, all women, include chairside assistants (5,600), secretary-receptionists (2,100), and dental technicians (1,600). There are only thirty dental hygienists, all attached to the armed services. Since 1975, however, the Department of Further Education, South

Australia, has conducted a one year course to train hygienists for hospital dental service and private practice.

School Dental Therapists

The fastest growing category of dental auxiliary is the operating school dental therapist, of whom there are now 400, some of them trained in New Zealand. Their number will increase even more rapidly in the future. When the decision was made to develop a national school dental scheme, Australia had two state run training schools, located in Tasmania and South Australia. Since then, nine additional State Health Department run schools have opened, and dental therapists are being recruited and trained in all six states. The eleven schools have a capacity to graduate 390 annually. A similar course for dental therapists has been offered for the past five years by the Western Australian Institute of Technology, whose graduates are permitted by law to work for private dentists as well as in government service. Few therapists have gained employment in private practice, however; other states and the Australian Dental Association have been reluctant to extend the work of the therapist to the private patient.

The scope of activity of the dental therapist in Australia resembles that in New Zealand, except that Australian therapists are trained to take and interpret x-rays. The Australian auxiliary is under much closer dentist control than her New Zealand counterpart, however, as can be seen from the ratio of one dentist to eight therapists in Australia compared with one dentist to sixty nurses in New Zealand.

ABOUT THE AUTHOR

Dr. Richard Logan is director of the Division of Dental Health in the Department of Health, New Zealand. Prior to assuming these national responsibilities, he was principal dental officer for Auckland, New Zealand.

Dr. Logan received his B.D.S. degree at the University of New Zealand and a Doctor of Public Health degree at the University of Sydney, Australia. As a demonstration of the respect between the island nations, Dr. Logan has been made a fellow of the Royal Australian College of Dental Surgeons.

His present address is: Department of Health, P.O. Box 5013, Wellington, New Zealand.

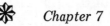 *Chapter 7*

Dental Care Delivery in Saskatchewan, Canada

Dr. Michael H. Lewis

Provincial Area: 655,200 square kilometers
    (Canada: 9,976,680 square kilometers)
Provincial Population: 926,000 (Canada: 23,100,000)
Per Capita Gross National Product: $6,190 (all Canada)
Life Expectancy: seventy-three years (all Canada)

There are about 214 dentists practicing in Canada's central prairie province of Saskatchewan, which gives a dentist to population ratio of 1:4,300. In Canada, one dentist serves approximately 3,024 people, so Saskatchewan is below the national average. Worse, half of the practicing dentists in Saskatchewan are located in the two major cities, Regina and Saskatoon, which have between them 30 percent of the total population. This means that the remaining 50 percent of dentists serve approximately 70 percent of the people of Saskatchewan, giving a dentist to population ratio of 1:7,000 for the small towns, villages, and isolated farms.

THE ORIGIN OF THE DENTAL NURSE PROGRAM FOR CHILDREN

Dental surveys conducted in 1968 showed that the dental health of the children in Saskatchewan was very poor. At age seven, children had an average of 5.4 primary teeth decayed, extracted, or filled. Of this number, more than three teeth per child were decayed while less than one was filled. Eleven year old children had an average of 2.3

decayed permanent teeth; 75 percent of these children needed fillings, and 26 percent needed extractions.

The poor dental health of children in the province, together with the serious shortage of dentists, caused the dental division of the Department of Health to seek alternative methods for delivering dental care to children. The division began with a pilot project in a rural area, which the federal government agreed to finance. In September 1970, a sixty-foot mobile home was converted into a four chair dental clinic to service, in rotation, four major elementary schools. A dentist was hired to supervise the project, and two dental auxiliaries from the "New Cross" School in London were hired to provide the dental care. At the end of two years, the project had demonstrated, first, that parents in rural Saskatchewan would enroll their children in a dental program where the basic services were provided by operating dental auxiliaries and, second, that the quality of care provided by the auxiliaries was considered satisfactory after regular examinations by a team of Saskatchewan private dental practitioners. On the basis of this successful project, the government of Saskatchewan in 1972 announced that a children's dental plan for the people of Saskatchewan would commence in two years.

Legislation was immediately passed to establish a training program in Regina for operating dental auxiliaries. The government decided that this dental auxiliary would be known as a Saskatchewan Dental Nurse, and the first thirty-six students were enrolled in the training program in the fall of 1972. The two year program is based on the New Zealand School Dental Nurse Program, but with greater emphasis on dental health education and disease prevention. Also, certain additional dental techniques are taught to the students, including the mandibular block injection, pulpotomies, and the placing of stainless steel crowns. By September 1976, one hundred students were enrolled—sixty for Saskatchewan and forty for the adjacent province of Manitoba, which is about to embark on a similar children's dental program.

Between 1972 and the commencement of the dental plan in September 1974, a great deal of planning and preparation was undertaken by the Dental Health Branch. For administrative purposes, the province was divided into six dental regions, averaging 160 kilometers by 110 kilometers. A town in each region was selected as a regional headquarter for an administrative officer, clerical staff, and an equipment maintenance technician.

It was decided that children would be phased into the program over a six year period, as shown in Figure 7−1. At the present time, five groups of children, covering ages five through nine, are enrolled.

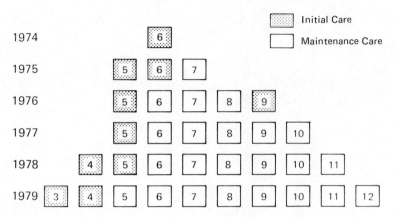

Figure 7—1. Phase-in Schedule—Dental Care over Six Year Period for Saskatchewan School Children, ages Three through Twelve.

In the following two school years, 1977–1979, it is anticipated that all children between the ages of three and twelve will be eligible for enrollment.

THE FIRST THREE YEARS

There are a total of 71,527 children now eligible for enrollment. Of these, 58,659, or 82.0 percent, are enrolled in the plan; 4,960, or 6.9 percent, have refused; and no response has been received from 7,908, or 11.1 percent (Table 7—1). We assume that the refusals represent parents whose children are established with a family dentist and are receiving regular dental care. Thus, we are more concerned about the 11 percent of children whose parents did not respond to the invitation to enroll, for we believe they will be equally disinterested in dental health and, therefore, that their children may be in great need of this program.

Staff

Dental services in the program are provided by dentists, dental nurses, and dental assistants. The dentists examine newly enrolled children, diagnose, plan treatment, and supervise an average of eight dental nurse teams each. Supervision consists of quality control of the work of the dental nurse, instruction in areas in which the dental nurse is weak or is having difficulty, ensuring that the work load of the region is completed on time, and also providing some clinical services beyond the competence of the dental nurse. During the first year of the program, the dentists spent a great deal of time on the

Table 7–1.   Saskatchewan Dental Plan Enrollment as of March 31, 1977. *(An encouraging average enrollment of 82 percent is abridged by the disappointing 11 percent of children whose parents did not respond to the invitation.)*

Year of Birth	Number Eligible	Enrolled	Percent	Refusal	Percent	No Response	Percent
1967	14,323	10,501	73.3	1,263	8.8	2,559	17.9
1968	13,982	12,368	88.5	666	4.8	948	6.8
1969	14,281	12,059	84.4	1,028	7.2	1,194	8.4
1970	14,146	12,034	85.1	933	6.6	1,179	8.3
1971	14,250	11,152	78.3	1,070	7.5	2,028	14.2
Other ages	545	545	100.0	—	—	—	—
Total:	71,527	58,659	82.0	4,960	6.9	7,908	11.1

road traveling between the various teams. Each dentist drove approximately 27,000 kilometers during the 1974–1975 school year. As more children are phased into the program, this travel time is decreasing, allowing the dentist to spend more of his time in dental clinics with the dental nurse teams.

The dental nurses provide classroom dental health instruction, chairside dental health instruction, prophylaxis, and application of topical fluoride, restorative services (using local anesthesia), and surgical services. Dental nurses are allowed to extract only primary teeth.

Dental assistants provide chairside dental health education, prophylaxis, and topical fluorides; expose and develop dental radiographs; provide chairside assistance; and also transport children from schools without clinics to the nearest school with a clinic.

Site Selection

It was decided early on that the dental services would be provided in the elementary schools. Because of a declining school population, most schools had space available that could readily be turned into a dental clinic. It was also recognized that the key to getting high enrollment in a dental program is to place the dental clinic as close to the children as possible, eliminating the need for parents to bring the children to the clinic and also eliminating the need for making firm appointments. The Department of Education supported this concept, and by the end of the first year of the program, 215 clinics had been established in elementary schools. A further sixty clinics were established during the second year, and we expect an additional sixty during 1977.

The area selected varied from an empty classroom to an infrequently used home economics room or space shared with the school public health nurse. Frequently, part of the room was used for other purposes, such as general school storage or office space, or as a remedial reading room. The lighting in the selected space usually had to be improved and additional utility electric outlets provided. A kitchen type sink with locking cupboards was placed on one wall, and an air compressor was placed in the boiler room with an air line to the clinic. We tried to ensure that 12.2 square meters of space were available for a dental clinic. The average cost to upgrade this space in the school during the first year of the program was approximately $2,500, not including dental equipment. Renovation costs are now $7,500, due to inflation and the more complex nature of renovations that are required in the remaining schools. These clinics are equipped with one dental chair, a mobile dental unit, a mobile cabinet, and two stools.

Many professional dental organizations originally suggested that the dental plan should operate through large dental clinics located around the province, with a staff of ten to twenty dental nurses and with children bussed in from surrounding schools; this, it was suggested, would prove more efficient and would allow over the shoulder supervision by a dentist. On investigation it was found that to feed a clinic of this size, the average busing distance in most of the province would be 56 kilometers and as much as 120 kilometers for some areas. Therefore, the concept was rejected. As an experiment, however, one ten-chair dental clinic has been built in a city where, because of expanding employment in the lumber industry, the elementary schools had no free space. Children from all the city schools, as well as the surrounding areas, are bussed into this clinic.

After two years' experience, we believe that one chair dental clinics established in as many schools as possible represent a better delivery system for us. The multiple chair clinic causes difficulties in appointment scheduling and also disrupts the schools. It becomes harder to involve parents in their children's dental care, and it is more upsetting for small children to have a bus journey followed by a visit to this large, slightly overwhelming dental clinic. We have also found dental nurses to be quite capable of working without the constant presence of a dentist. In fact, they respond very well to the challenge.

Equipment and Supplies

The equipment used is standard throughout the program (Table 7–2). Where possible, it is made so it can be readily moved out if, because of a declining school population, we decide to close a clinic. Equipment includes a basic, electrically operated contour dental chair with a post-mounted light; we have avoided the hydraulic-based chair because of the weight factor and also to eliminate the possibility of oil spillage. The basic dental unit is an Adec modification of the Micro-cart 3, selected because of its portability and the lack of plumbing required. The unit carries its own water system, three way syringe, a high and low speed handpiece, high volume suction, and a saliva ejector; to operate, it is only necessary to make a quick connection to an air line. The unit is usually placed on the assistant's side of the chair, and the top is used as a work surface. Each permanent clinic has a mobile cabinet for storage of dental supplies.

We have a number of portable dental x-rays that fit into a bracket mounted on the clinic wall. The position of the bracket has to be ap-

Table 7–2. Equipment Purchased for Permanent and Portable Clinics—Saskatchewan Dental Plan, August 1976.

Equipment Item	Number per Clinic	Manufacturer (model)	Cost per Clinic
(a) Permanent Clinic			
Total:			$4,897.97
Air compressor	1	Webster (402-3)	525.00
Amalgamator*	1	Toothmaster (300)	68.78
Dental chair (fixed)	1	Vacudent (P-60-AIBS)	1,156.60
Dental light (fixed)	1	Pelton and Crane (Light Fantastic)	245.70
Dental cabinet	1	Denco (7 drawer)	176.32
Dental unit*	1	Adec (Sask–Cart)	696.86
Autoclave (chemiclave)*	1	Harvey (4000)	292.68
X-ray machine*	1	Siemens (Heliodent 60)	1,417.50
X-ray developer*	1	Procomat (II)	197.40
Dental stools (portable)*	2	Office Specialty (708M)	94.72
Dental x-ray viewer*	1	Illuminator (14 1/8 × 5 3/8)	26.41
(b) Portable Clinic			
Total:			$3,679.49
Air compressor	1	Scripline (¾ HP Motor, 6 gallon tank)	415.28
Amalgamator*	1	Toothmaster (300)	68.78
Dental chair (portable)	1	Adec (c/w Light Post)	272.40
Dental light (portable)	1	Roland (Fibreoptic)	197.46
Dental unit*	1	Adec (Sask–Cart)	696.86
Autoclave (chemiclave)*	1	Harvey (4000)	292.68
X-ray machine*	1	Siemens (Heliodent 60)	1,417.50
X-ray developer*	1	Procomat (II)	197.40
Dental stools (portable)*	2	Office Specialty (708M)	94.72
Dental x-ray viewer*	1	Illuminator (14 1/8 × 5 3/8)	26.41

*These items are common to both permanent and portable clinics and need not be duplicated except in situations where they may be required in two different locations simultaneously.

Source: Annual Report, Saskatchewan Dental Plan, 1976.

proved by the radiation health officer of the Occupational Health Branch, and we are not allowed to use mobile stands. The x-ray separates into two parts, so it can be carried from one clinic to another by the dental nurse team. We use an automatic processor for developing the x-rays, thus eliminating the need for a darkroom.

If we have space available in a school but the enrollment does not warrant establishing a permanent dental clinic, the dental nurse team provides care using portable equipment. Portable equipment consists of an instrument case and a folding dental chair with a fibroptic light mounted on it. The same basic dental unit is used in both permanent and portable clinics, as it can readily be placed in the back of a station wagon and transported from one clinic to another, along with a portable compressor to supply air to run the unit (see Table 7—2). (When possible, because of the noise, we place the compressor in an adjoining room and run a flexible airhose to the unit.)

To serve the very remote areas of the province where schools are very small—sometimes with only half a dozen pupils—we have equipped two motor homes as dental clinics. These are eight and one half meter Champion Units, each fitted with two dental chairs, its own compressor, and electrical generator.

While the concept of these motor homes is wonderful, we have found them to have serious limitations in Saskatchewan (see also Chapter 15, on Norway). The weather is too cold for them to be used during the severe winter months. Even though they are winterized, there are real problems, because of freezing, in taking on water and getting rid of wastes. Most of these remote areas are served by narrow gravel roads, and it is a real challenge to drive an eight and one-half meter wide mobile home into some of these schools when the roads are icy and snow clogged. In addition, we have found that most Saskatchewan school playgrounds are anything but level, and the unit must first be leveled with jacks. All in all, these units have not been very satisfactory. They are excellent for doing surveys and for working during the spring, summer, and fall months, but for five months of the year they are totally unsuitable. We have found that it is better, during the winter months, for a dental nurse team with a station wagon and a portable dental chair to handle these small schools.

All supplies for the dental plan are purchased centrally. We have our own warehouse in Regina for storage and shipping. After two years, we are improving our stock control procedures in order to get the best bulk prices without carrying an excessively large stock on hand; thus, we equalize the cash flow for the operation and assist the supplier by not purchasing a year's supply in one shipment. We also have our own repair depot and maintain and service all the dental equipment either in the field or in the warehouse. Our chief technician has visited all the factories of our suppliers of dental equipment and is able to make major repairs, thus eliminating the need to send faulty equipment back to the factory.

Costs

The program is totally financed from general provincial revenue. There are no premiums or fees of any kind levied against the users of this program. To equalize the cash flow over the initial five years of operation, most of the major capital equipment was purchased during the first year of the program when staff numbers were low.

The actual costs for the first two years of operation, including depreciation of fixed assets at a rate of 15 percent, are shown in Table 7—3. It should be noted that the cost per child was reduced by $50 in the second year, from $158 to $107. This compares with a cost of $116 per child if the services are costed out using the fee schedule of the Saskatchewan College of Dental Surgeons. During this same period, there was a 20 percent increase in salaries of dental nurses and dental assistants. I anticipate that the cost per child will fall to about $95 in 1976.* Dental nurses have increased their productivity, so that they are now treating, on average, 510 children per nurse. Planning calls for each dental nurse to treat about 580 children next year.

Table 7—3. Saskatchewan Dental Plan—Two Year Cost of Service. *(The dramatic 50 percent drop in cost per child is expected to fall an additional 11 percent in 1976. This decrease in cost is in spite of 20 percent wage increase.)*

	Program Year September 1974— August 1975	Program Year September 1975— August 1976
Actual cost of services	$2,079,968	$4,052,293
Number of enrolled children	13,140	37,571
Average cost per enrolled child	$158	$107

*Third year costs actually dropped to $83 per child in 1976, a 22.4 percent decrease from 1975 and an overall decrease of $75 or 48 percent from the first year.

A breakdown of the $107 cost per child in 1975–1976 is as follows:

Salaries	$70.53
Travel, hotel, sustenance	9.74
Dental supplies	5.07
Depreciation	4.68
Other	16.98

EVALUATION TO DATE

The dental health of the children enrolled in the program is shown in Table 7–4. Statistics for the children born in 1968 should reflect children on maintenance care, but they are distorted by 1,200 children born in 1968 but newly enrolled in the second year of the program. The ratio of filled deciduous and permanent teeth to DMF + DEF for all those born in 1968 is 53 percent. Had it been possible to isolate the statistics of the children born in 1968 who were on maintenance care, however, I believe this figure would have increased to 70 or 80 percent. As is evident, children born in 1969 and 1970 reflect the poor health found in surveys before the program started. Thus, it is of doubtful value to try to measure the effect of the program by examining statistics during the early years of the dental program. Rather, it is necessary to look at the actual services provided.

There are also less tangible benefits that I have noticed more and more as I visit clinics around the province. I have noticed that children are coming down to the dental nurse clinics during recess on days when it is too cold to go outdoors. I have seen as many as fifteen kids hanging over the chair, watching the dental nurse restore a tooth, touching instruments, blowing air, and generally interfering with the best sterile techniques. At first, I was horrified. But then I decided that maybe this was the best dental health education we could provide. Children were going down to see their friend, the dental nurse; they trusted her. There was obviously no fear, and more importantly, they were really understanding something about dental health and the importance of preventing dental decay. These are perhaps the most important lessons we can teach the children.

Quality Evaluation

At the end of the program's first year, it was felt that there must be a more formal evaluation of the Saskatchewan Dental Plan. It was decided, therefore, to evaluate and compare the quality of amalgam

Table 7–4. Dental Health of Enrolled Children, Saskatchewan Dental Plan, September 1974 to August 1975 and September 1975 to August 1976.

| | Average Number Per Child | | | |
| Dental Health Indicators | September 1974–August 1975 | September 1975–August 1976 by Year of Birth | | |
		1968	1969	1970
Decayed, extracted, filled—deciduous teeth (DEF)	5.61	5.51	5.56	4.94
Decayed	4.11	1.58	3.89	3.88
Extracted	0.44	0.72	0.46	0.25
Filled	1.06	3.20	1.19	0.79
Decayed, missing, filled—permanent teeth (DMF)	0.94	1.95	0.80	0.15
Decayed	0.90	1.13	0.73	0.13
Extracted	0.00	0.02	0.01	0.00
Filled	0.04	0.79	0.06	0.01
Total DEF + DMF	6.55	7.47	6.36	5.09
Percent of filled deciduous and permanent teeth to DMF + DEF	17	53	19	15

Source: Annual Reports, Saskatchewan Plan.

Table 7−5. Comparative Quality of Amalgam Restorations Placed
by Saskatchewan Dental Nurses and Dentists.

Number of Restorations	Dentists 604	Dental Nurses 1,503
	(percentage)	
Unacceptable	21.1	3.7
Adequate	62.4	48.6
Superior	16.5	47.7

and stainless steel crown restorations provided by the dental nurse,
on the one hand, and dentists in private practice, on the other. Three
dentists—a pedodontist and two restorative specialists—surveyed 410
children in Grades I and II. A blind technique was used so that the
examiners could not tell which operator type had performed the
treatment. A total of 2,107 amalgam restorations and 97 stainless
steel crowns were assessed. Overall, the amalgam restorations were
rated as shown in Table 7−5. A breakdown of these findings according to one- or multisurface restorations, in deciduous or permanent
teeth, showed that the Saskatchewan dental nurse placed amalgam
fillings that, on average, were better than those placed by dentists.
There was no quality difference between the performance by dentists
and that by dental nurses with respect to stainless steel crowns.

PROFESSIONAL REACTION

The reaction of the private dental community in Saskatchewan to
the dental program—apart from the aforementioned minor embar-
rassment—is interesting. Initially, dentists were fearful. They asked
questions like, What are your dental nurses going to do when a patient goes into anaphylactic shock? But what they were really asking,
I believe, was, What is this program going to do to my practice?
Three years have passed now, and the College of Dental Surgeons of
Saskatchewan supports the dental program. There are certain aspects
of which they are critical, but generally they support it. And I think
the reasons are quite obvious. Private dentists are busier than ever
before. Their income in the two and a half years the program has
been operating has increased by $10,000 net (from an average of
$30,519 in 1973). The pattern of practice has also changed. Gener-
ally, dentists are not treating many children any more. But they are
providing more, and more sophisticated, dental care to adults. Many
more crowns and bridges are being provided and, in general, a great
deal more of the sort of dentistry that results in greater income.

In the rest of Canada, there is still much opposition to the Saskatchewan Dental Plan, particularly from the province of Ontario, where dentists in certain areas are in oversupply. In Saskatchewan, where there is more demand for dentistry than can be handled, many of the initial concerns of the profession are no longer voiced.

Thus, even without detailed statistical evidence, I believe this program must be considered a success. It is most suitable for the particular situation in Saskatchewan and, I believe, for many areas where there is a scattered rural population and a shortage of dentists. But it obviously cannot be transplanted wholesale to other areas where the same conditions do not prevail.

ABOUT THE AUTHOR

Dr. Michael Lewis is director of the Saskatchewan dental plan in the Saskatchewan Department of Health. Prior to assuming the directorship of the Saskatchewan Dental Nurse Program, Dr. Lewis was a regional dental health officer in Saskatchewan. Previously, he practiced general dentistry in Kelowna, British Columbia.

Dr. Lewis is English by birth and was an officer in the British Army before immigrating to Canada. He received his D.D.S. degree from the University of Alberta and a doctorate in Dental Public Health from the University of Toronto.

His present address is: Saskatchewan Dental Plan, 3211 Albert Street, Regina, Saskatchewan.

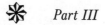 *Part III*

Innovative Programs
from the Americas

Clearly, a good deal of the credit must go to the Pan American Health Organization for the changes in dental care delivery occurring in the Americas. On the other hand, none of these accomplishments would have been possible were it not for the interested and enlightened governments and concerned members of the profession who became involved.

The movement for change is more widespread than these selected studies indicate. Jamaica and Trinidad, for example, are developing expanded duty auxiliaries to broaden the base of care.

Most noteworthy in these reports is the unusual involvement of the local communities. As Dr. George Gillespie points out (Chapter 9), community involvement "does not refer merely to calling community leaders to the dental or administrative offices to discuss provisions of the dental services; it means going out into the community and discussing matters of dental care, matters of daily life, and aspects of the community's own economy. . . . It is necessary to change the system and radically change the system of delivery."

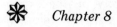 *Chapter 8*

Dental Care Delivery in the State of Mexico

Dr. Gustavo Baz Diaz Lombardo

Area: 21,000 square kilometers
    (all Mexico: 1,960,000 square kilometers)
Population: 7,700,000 (all Mexico, 63,000,000)
Per Capita Gross National Product: $1,090 (all Mexico)
Life Expectancy: sixty-three years (all Mexico)

Until now, dentistry in Mexico has barely served to provide curative and restorative care to economically able social classes, with marginal attention to some other sectors, particularly labor. There are only 14,000 dentists in the entire country to care for a population of sixty-three million—a ratio of 1:4,500—and virtually no auxiliary dental personnel. In the state of Mexico, which surrounds the federal district (Mexico City), the ratio of dentists to population is far lower —1:15,400—evidence of the enormous disproportion between areas. It is estimated that some twenty million people in Mexico, three million of them in the state of Mexico, have no health care, much less dental care, on a permanent basis. The facts are that most of the population lacks dental care and that even what is available is not of the highest quality. Another complicating factor is that 62 percent of the population is urban, much of it in huge slums. The remaining 38 percent is dispersed in the countryside, often difficult to reach.

Part of this complex distribution is due to the dental schools, which perpetuate problems by turning out professionals who tend to work only for those members of the urban population who can pay. These dentists master a certain amount of restorative technology but have little capacity or desire to meet the needs of the great majority of the population; all too often, they rely on the expensive techniques and equipment found in more highly developed societies. Dental clinics for poor people in the cities and rural areas are scarce and often of inadequate quality; equally scarce are preventive action and education, as well as resources for research. In addition, Mexico's size, inadequate communications network, maldistribution of income, and low educational status all contribute to the inaccessibility of dental care. Even so, the availability of dentists for routine care of oral disease is unequal to demand, as overcrowded waiting rooms testify. Professionals in both public and private facilities are required to work long hours.

In a developing country, it is slow and difficult work to establish a dental delivery system, even for those of a high economic stratum. In Mexico, and in developing countries generally, equipment maintenance is extremely costly, due to distances from population centers, high importing costs, unavailability of spare parts, and a shortage of skilled technicians. By contrast, in developed countries, the cost, maintenance, and updating of equipment are within easy reach of professionals, enabling them to remain up to the minute. Another deterrent to progress in developing countries is the delay in communication of recent advances in research and the fact that most professionals have no funds to attend informative events, which usually take place outside the country.

THE PILOT PROGRAM IN NEZAHUALCOYOTL CITY

This lack of human resources, their poor geographical distribution, the fact that only the wealthier classes have access to health care (basically of a curative nature), and the restricted availability of financial resources have led us, in the state of Mexico, to explore other avenues to achieve a more forceful impact on the population's health. Our motto is: *Nobody will come to solve our problems. We have to solve them by ourselves.*

The first priority has been to make public health the joint action of professionals and the society in which they live. Thus, while the state health council directs health care delivery, a member of the health services, appointed by the local municipal council, is given the responsibility of developing health programs in conjunction with the community, with the aim of attaining higher productivity and greater coverage.

Our first program was initiated in 1973 in Nezahualcoyotl City, one of the most densely populated marginal settlements in the state of Mexico. The city abounds in all the urban problems generated by the inflow of peasants and the unemployed so common in Latin American cities.

In Nezahualcoyotl City, for the past three years, one stomatological care module has been an integral part of the city's health system, which also includes a general hospital, seven health care centers, three child care centers, and one sanitary control center. Financing for this system comes from both federal and state governments and is managed by the State Public Health Coordinated Services Bureau. The system delivers medical and dental care, carries out preventive work, has a community health education project, conducts sociological and epidemiological investigations, and provides a growing source of employment and health training for community residents.

Medical and Community Services

The system is enormously helped by the one year public health residency for newly graduated physicians, which was created in an attempt to relieve the economic and geographical maldistribution of health personnel. For six straight hours every day during the course of one year, these public health residents examine, diagnose, and treat those who come to the health centers for care. (Difficult cases are referred to the general hospital.)

Medical practice in the health center is combined with work in the community, where physicians provide health education and promote the creation of discussion groups to extend the Health Ministry's epidemiological control programs. The doctors also investigate community problems, correlating theory with practice. In the future, personnel with this solid training in the realities of Mexican urban life will better serve the state of Mexico's expanding public health network.

Auxiliaries

The Public Health Coordinated Services Bureau is supplementing these doctors with its own programs for training health technicians from among the local community. It conducts a one year course for these special auxiliaries (ages sixteen to twenty) that includes both course work—in basic biomedical and health subjects, knowledge of local conditions and problems, and work methodology—and field work. Every morning for twelve months, the trainees work intensively in all preventive medical campaigns, going door to door. They take part in health education courses, family planning, vaccination, and general health promotion. Thus, the health care network is being expanded even as more personnel are trained and more local people employed.

Young women who have already finished secondary school (ninth grade) are enrolled in the local nursing school, while others are being trained as clinical nurses aides. Some nurses aides learn to become "clinical dental technicians," who provide primary care, under the supervision of a dentist, for children who come to the stomatological care center. They also teach them nutrition and oral hygiene.

DENTAL SERVICE

A new stomatologic practice system is being developed to serve as a model for dental care for the state of Mexico and eventually for the entire nation. Making use of what we learned in Nezahualcoyotl City, we are proposing a system of regional centers to serve large urban communities as well as to handle referrals from their outlying areas. Additional arrangements are made for rural areas.

The system will have four basic services—(1) stationary stomatological care modules in urban centers; (2) similar but lighter and more mobile geodesic dome units in well-populated rural areas; (3) home-to-home care in sparsely settled rural areas; and (4) specialist services provided on referral from the other three services. The program budget for the five year period 1976—1980 is approximately $5,425,000, growing toward an annual expenditure of $1,340,000 and a coverage of 200,000 people by 1980.

Urban Stomatological Care
Modules (stationary)

Related to the health centers and as part of the overall health system, a model stationary stomatological care module that consists of two prefabricated fiberglass sections has been built in Nezahualcoyotl City. One section serves as an administration and waiting room area. The other section is the clinical area, with nine locally manufactured dental chairs grouped around a central service island. At each chair, using four-handed techniques, a clinical dental technician and a clinical assistant deliver basic dental care to children. The mouth is treated by quadrants under local anesthesia. No more than five appointments complete full mouth treatment. From the central island, an assistant prepares work trays and hands the operating teams the supplies they require. X-ray equipment is also available.

The entire operation of the stationary stomatological care module is supervised by a dentist, who is also responsible for diagnosis and treatment plans and acts in situations for which the auxiliary and technical staff are not trained.

Twenty-three persons staff the stationary module. They are:

Dentist	1
Clinical Technicians	9
Clinical Assistants	11
Administrative Officer	1
Transportation Officer	1

Using this mix of personnel, a more productive job, of better quality and training value, and at a lower unit cost, is done.

The waiting room unit of the stationary dental care module serves as a classroom as well. Here, children either have classes with their regular teachers or receive education in nutrition and oral hygiene from the staff while waiting their turn. Buses are used to bring children from school as their treatment is programmed.

We have found that, with community education, there is a growing demand for dental services, even though each child is required to pay something (10 pesos, or about 40 cents) per treatment for basic dental care. The average cost of basic dental care is 153 pesos (a little under $7) per child per year, and it is expected that 7,000 children will be treated annually. The cost per center is:

Operating (annual)	$78,762
Capital Investment	$56,785

Concentrated Rural Areas

For well-populated areas, we have designed clinics of a lightweight structure, known as *Tetra Hidros*, that are basically similar to those used in urban centers except that there are only six chairs instead of nine. These units are prefabricated geodesic domes with metal ribs and plastic reinforced panels mounted on a cement base. These domes can be transported by trucks and reassembled as needed. They are self-contained units with their own power generators, water, and air compressors and can be assembled or taken down in two or three hours by people with no special training. It is particularly important that this be done by people from the community, both to provide needed employment and to interest them in the oral health system. In appearance, the *Tetra Hidro* clinic is light and attractive and not at all intimidating to the children who come for treatment.

The program remains in a community from six to twelve months, depending on the size of the community. Children are treated at the modules, which also act as home base for dentally equipped jeeps traveling into the countryside. The auxiliary personnel are trained on site, and when the program is moved to another place, these auxiliaries stay in their own community, promoting oral health and maintaining education in dental hygiene and the basics of dental health.

The basic staff of sixteen for the concentrated rural clinic consists of:

Dentist	1
Clinical Technicians	6
Assistants	7
Administrative Officer	1
Transportation Officer	1

We expect to cover 6,300 children per clinic per year under this program. The cost per center is:

Operating (annual)	$58,416
Capital Investment	$43,480

Home-to-Home Care in Remote Areas

In more sparsely settled areas, care is delivered on a home-to-home basis, thus covering the entire family. Trucks and jeeps set out from the "home base" *Tetra Hidro* facilities to deliver dental care to the most remote places. The trucks can transport an average of ten units (each with one chair), but where access is more difficult, jeeps carry one or two units. All systems employ simplified equipment, which is absolutely self-contained and mounted in special cases for transportation.

Each rural unit is operated by one clinical technician and one assistant. Personnel use the minimum necessary instruments and simplified techniques to provide basic care. They spend much time gaining the confidence of the general population as well as community leaders in order to leave behind better oral health procedures after they move on. Expected coverage is 1,200 persons per jeep per year. The cost (per jeep) is:

Operating (annual)	$6,800
Capital Investment	$2,800

Specialist Services

From all clinics or treatment teams, complex cases and complications are referred to hospital centers, where specialists and adequate equipment are available to handle problems in any area of stomatology. In addition, we expect to build specialist centers with offices for outpatient consultations and rooms for simple surgery not requiring an operating room. The first of these will specialize in maxillofacial surgery, with one specialist, a maxillofacial surgery resident, and a staff of two clinical assistants. The cost per year of each maxillofacial center is about $18,650, with a coverage of 400 persons per team.

ELEMENTS OF THE NEW PHILOSOPHY

The program outlined above is bringing stomatological care to people who have never before received it. We can do this because we are making use of all of the following human resources to take the place of, reinforce, and improve the work formerly done by a single person —the dentist.

1. In order to optimize *local community* involvement in the programs, we are using attractive booklets that are easy to read to guide the people toward health services. For those who have little opportunity to read or are illiterate, pictures are used.
2. With simple training, *natural leaders* can organize their communities and provide both preventive and curative guidance.
3. *Auxiliary personnel*, basically composed of newly trained persons from the community itself, become part of the official oral care delivery system.
4. In addition, *laboratory and clinical technical staff* work in specific areas under the supervision of stomatologists.
5. *Stomatologists*, in turn, work in areas that require deeper knowledge and act as leaders of the oral health team.

CONCLUSIONS

Thus, the stomatological programs currently under way in the state of Mexico reflect a new approach to care in marginal communities, new kinds of personnel training, and new ways to reach the public in need of dental care. This approach is beginning to gain acceptance at some universities, such as the Universidad Autonoma Metropolitana and E.N.E.P., Zaragoza, at least to the extent that dentists are being taught the value of working in teams with auxiliaries and the importance of extending prevention and care to wider elements in the population.

Private dentists attacked the program in the past, but their antagonism diminished as they realized we are working with people who cannot pay private dentists anyway.

We believe that our program represents an important step in the search for extending good quality stomatological care to all individuals and communities in our state and that it will contribute to the design of systems with the same goals all over Latin America.

ABOUT THE AUTHOR

Dr. Gustavo Baz, a physician, is presently the chief of the Coordinated Public Health Services for the state of Mexico. Prior to that he was director of the health system of the city of Nezahualcoyotl. He has also served as the chief of surgery at the Central Medical Center and concurrently as professor of surgery at the National Autonomous University of Mexico where he graduated with an M.D. degree in 1958. Dr. Baz received his advanced surgical training at the University of Minnesota, Minneapolis.

His present address is: Avenida Cuauhtemoc 28, San Jeronimo Licide, Mexico, D.F.

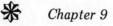 *Chapter 9*

Dental Care Delivery in Venezuela

Dr. George M. Gillespie

Area: 911,680 square kilometers
Population: 12,000,000
Per Capita Gross National Product: $2,037
Life Expectancy: sixty-four years

Over the past five years, some exciting experiments in delivery of dental care have been put into place in Venezuela. Since it is a developing country, Venezuela has a certain freedom to select new directions, but its experiences might have implications even for new approaches to be considered in the United States. As the discussion on Ecuador suggests, (see Chapter 10), other countries in Latin America are already building on the Venezuelan experience.

SOME HISTORY

In 1966, there were only 1,500 dentists in the whole of Venezuela. The dentist to population ratio was 1:5,400 in metropolitan areas, 1:10,000 in other urban areas, and a dramatic 1:75,000 in the countryside. Only sixteen institutions were providing dental care, seven on a national basis and nine at the local level. It had been estimated that by the time Venezuelans reached the age of twenty, six out of ten of their teeth were affected by caries. Rural children were virtually unattended. These imbalances reflect similar imbalances throughout the Venezuelan national picture. Whereas the average annual per capita income of $2,057 is relatively high for Latin America, it has been estimated that 80 percent of the population receives less than $250 per head. Seventy-five percent of the population is crowded into Caracas and a handful of other cities.

This situation was cause for concern in dentistry as elsewhere, and in this context the Ministry of Development, together with the professional associations and the Ministry of Health, decided to undertake a survey of dental care facilities, dental schools, and dental care needs. Some 32,000 household interviews were conducted in eighty counties, and clinical examinations were made of about 6,000 people, based on a national sample. The ministry sought to answer such questions as what types and numbers of dentists were required for Venezuela; what was the role of the faculties of dentistry; how could urban–rural maldistribution be overcome; what sort of practice patterns should be promoted; and what types of auxiliaries should be produced, if any?

The survey indicated that fourteen year olds exhibited a DMF rate of 7.4, with only 12 percent of the carious lesions showing signs of restoration. Sixty-five percent of the population, and a relatively higher proportion among lower income groups, showed signs of periodontal disease. As for the limited dental care that was being done, 57 percent was being provided by private practice, only 34 percent by public institutions, and the remainder by charitable or other bodies. Only 24 percent of private practice was being devoted to people with less than $300 annual income. The public sector was providing the major share (86 percent) of what little dental care was reaching the rural areas.

Based on these observations, it was determined that an experimental area would be developed in which some hypotheses could be tested and new solutions sought while the original data were being analyzed. The University of Zulia, whose dental faculty at Maracaibo is the second largest in Venezuela, was selected to take the lead. The idea was to develop an educational system that would be integrated with a service system operated by the faculty of dentistry. With the backing of the Ministry of Health and technical assistance from PAHO/WHO, a plan was developed in conjunction with the university. The latter initiated the program in 1969 with its own funds and local community support. Modifications were made within the faculty structure to set up a Department of Preventive Dentistry that would assume responsibility, including financial responsibility, for the programs. As the programs became established, local authorities provided funds from local and state budgets to continue and expand them.

NEW APPROACHES TO DENTAL CARE

After consulting with communities selected through a sample of the national survey, the dental faculty at Zulia made plans to open five clinics—or community laboratories, as they are called—in a four state area. As Table 9—1 shows, each clinic served an area with different demographic characteristics, though none was more than an eleven hour drive from Maracaibo. Clinics have been operating in the first four areas for some years. In each community, the local administration was required to give evidence of interest by, for example, donating a facility to house the clinic. The clinic projected for Maracaibo has not yet opened, due mainly to the need for additional financing.

When this program began, it was essential to think of more appropriate ways to reach the local population, as well as to know the cultural patterns and attitudes of the people to be involved. Consequently, dental staff associated with the new clinics took time to visit families wherever they were located. Surveys were developed in conjunction with a sociologist to ascertain community ideas about dental health and to get some impressions as to income and the stability of income, shopping habits, and sources of services. This way of involving the community clearly resulted in greater community interest once the clinics were opened.

Dental students were an integral part of the new program. In order to promote social awareness, the university required all students to spend their last year almost entirely outside the school of dentistry. They had to live in each community for at least six weeks, rotate through the different kinds of community experiences, and be responsible for their own food, housing, and participation in the community. Under faculty supervision, the students carried out the community surveys and undertook preliminary clinical examinations. Once the clinics were opened, a supervisor conducted inservice education programs in conjunction with the student clinical performance. Students were exposed to all phases of the system, including responsibility for administration, patient complaints, and other problems. One can see the impact of the community experience on the finished graduates. They are much more capable of producing dental care for the population at large than those who graduate from a traditional school.

The community surveys uncovered a clear need for specific dental services, such as the provision of dental prostheses. Seventy-six percent of the population examined needed tooth replacement—the sad

Table 9-1. University of Zulia Community Laboratories.

Community	State	Demography	Population	Status
			(total/children)	
El Pedregal	Falcon	rural village (concentrated)	2,200/500	opened 1970
San Felipe	Yaracuy	urban	43,000/10,000	opened 1971
San Francisco	Lara	urban (marginal)	17,095/3,946	opened 1972
El Guanabano	Zulia	rural (dispersed)	1,050/n.a.	opened 1971
Maracaibo	Zulia	metropolitan	600,000/n.a.	not yet opened

Source: PAHO.

end of a traditional relief of pain service involving an occasional visit to the dentist for extractions. In addition to an improved system for providing relief of pain services, there was a need to provide greater emphasis on preventive and restorative care.

Since part of the idea was to look for new approaches to the use of auxiliaries, it was necessary to break down auxiliary personnel functions beyond the "classic" categories of dental hygienist, dental assistant, and dental nurse. An analysis of tasks identified some thirty-five functions that local high school age girls could be trained to perform. Training objectives were identified for each of these functions, and training programs were set up. It was evident very soon that enough people would be willing to participate.

The auxiliaries were trained very efficiently and effectively, some to a level of New Zealand dental nurses and in a considerably shorter period of time. They were rapidly incorporated into the intensive dental health education program for school children, to teach such basic functions as tooth brushing and oral hygiene. It is worth noting that, in a matter of three to four weeks, these girls became extremely efficient in chairside assisting; in fact, they may now be proving to be the best teachers to instruct dental students in four-handed dentistry.

One of the problems faced was to break down the traditional barrier between the intramural faculty and the extramural experience. In the university clinic, students had been working under intense supervision, with traditional equipment and no chairside assistance; they were being trained to provide mainly a classic one chair–one operator relief of pain service. Now they were being exposed to working with auxiliaries and performing sitdown dentistry. In virtually the same space normally used by the old health clinic system, a team was now able to work under the supervision of a dentist and coordinated by dental students. The student reaction was notable. In a very short time, they demanded that equipment at the university clinics correspond more to present-day dentistry, with anatomic style chairs and other modern and functional equipment. Clinics in the faculty of dentistry, Maracaibo, have now been remodeled.

A major barrier to the implementation of rural health programs has been the difficulty of providing suitable low cost equipment and the expense of traditional equipment. Because of its extramural program, the faculty at Zulia has been forced to establish criteria for such equipment and to develop a capacity to produce it. With the aid of the university faculty of engineering, simplified dental equipment has been developed that has the same function as most of the imported equipment used previously. A simple dental chair made in the faculty of engineering costs about $200 to manufacture. The elimination of such unnecessary elements as water heaters for dental units and vertical movement in dental chairs has also helped to reduce costs. A rural clinic can now be established in a very short period of time at a minimum cost.

EXPERIENCE IN THE CLINICS

The first community laboratory was opened in 1970 in El Pedregal. In the early days, there was intense community interest and participation. A system of payment was devised that enabled a large percentage of the village to afford dental care. The system was based on fee for service, but with fees defined in a special way. The survey conducted at the beginning of the program had identified three predominant income ranges, and three corresponding fee schedules were developed. Sixty percent of the population received service under one or another of the basic fee schedules in the first years. An increase in the permitted length of payment time brought a further 10 percent into the clinic, a small subsidy increased coverage by another 5.0 percent, and an intensive education program to reach those who weren't coming to the clinic increased coverage by another 10 percent. Thus, 85 percent of the population has been covered at one time or another.

Gradually, however, as more of the population came under a maintenance system, patient attendance has tended to decrease. Services were provided to only about 20 percent of the community in 1976, compared to around 60 percent in 1972. Another community factor may have influenced the drop in attendance: El Pedregal benefited considerably from the national attention it received because of the new dental program. It now has water, lights, industry, and a thriving small economy based on the manufacture of hammocks. Some elements in the community evidently feared that the very success of the laboratory program in dramatically decreasing the need for restorative care might also cause the program to be terminated and permit El Pedregal to revert to its past isolation—a pattern that is all too familiar in rural development programs in El Pedregal and elsewhere.

Participation in San Felipe, an urban center, has hovered around 20 percent. However, in San Francisco, a marginally urbanized community, one-third of the population has been served since April 1976.

Table 9–2 shows the 1976 distribution of service at three of the clinics opened thus far. In San Felipe, most patients are coming for fillings and other forms of maintenance care. The other clinics are still performing large numbers of extractions, reflecting the greater numbers of first time patients. Clearly, however, new ways need to

Table 9-2. Service Components at University of Zulia Clinics, 1976.

Clinic	Percentage of Population Served (adult/children)	Number of Treatments	First Appointment	Fillings (percent)	Extractions	Other
El Pedregal	19.5/22.4	3,306	24.7	31.7	35.1	8.5
San Felipe	17.6/23.8	19,092	19.7	56.4	8.6	15.3
San Francisco (9 months)	30.5/23.6	7,397	35.0	32.0	19.0	14.0

Source: PAHO.

be found to bring tooth replacement to the rural population; less than 2 percent of treatment at each clinic has involved dentures, although the baseline survey indicated that 70 percent of the adult population needed them. It has become apparent that the traditional system of five or six sittings to fit one denture is unacceptable for many people who must take time out from employment to visit the dentist and who may have problems of transportation to the dentist's office. It should be possible to work out a system whereby two or three stages can be completed in one visit, so that the patient need only come back for the finished product.

NATIONWIDE IMPACT

From the original experimental program started in 1970, these community-based programs have now spread throughout most of Venezuela, thanks to a national policy decision taken by the Ministry of Health with regard to the use of teams of professionals and auxiliaries in rural dental care programs. By 1977, fifty-seven rural programs had been developed by the Ministry of Health, with 795 dentists involved. A separate budget for dental health has been established at the national level, and the national investment in dentistry has been increased.

In place of the 1,500 dentists who were licensed previously, there are now 4,000. New graduates are not concentrating only in Caracas. Dental students who have graduated from the Zulia program are now practicing in areas where dentists would not have considered practicing earlier. And they have found that their incomes have not suffered; in fact, by setting the scale of fees according to the economy of their patients, some of them have more than doubled their incomes over those of previous graduates.

In urban areas, the dentist to population ratio has dropped from 1:5,400 to 1:3,000. The impact in rural areas is particularly dramatic; from a 1966 ratio of 1:75,000, the ratio has dropped to 1:13,000. In addition, there are now 1,200 auxiliaries working in the health care system. It is also interesting to note that students trained under the University of Zulia method are continuing to conduct local surveys of community needs when they establish their own practice.

State governments have begun active financial participation in the clinic programs. Indeed, the state of Falcon, where El Pedregal is located, has now begun a statewide system; it served 41,733 patients in 1976. Although dentists at the Falcon clinics were still making almost two extractions for every filling in 1976 (see Table 9–3),

Table 9–3.   Falcon State Dental Services, 1976.

Patients Served 41,733

Appointments
First Appointments 18,099
Total   30,264

Clinical Activities
Fillings   9,258 = 36.5
Extractions 16,082 = 63.5

Cost
Patient per Year   36.82 Bs.
Appointment per Year 54.78 Bs.

Source: PAHO.

they were increasing the number of completed treatments, particularly in children—and at an average cost of only $20 per child.

The University of Zulia program illustrates the impact a university can have on a dental care delivery system. There are many things still to be analyzed and many experiences to be reevaluated. But in the course of the past five years, the program has produced a noticeable difference in health care coverage, particularly for the rural populations of Venezuela.

There are some very clear lessons here. First, the community must be involved at the beginning. This does not refer merely to calling community leaders to the dental or administrative office to discuss provision of dental services; it means going out into the community and discussing matters of dental care, matters of daily life, and aspects of the community's own economy. Another important lesson is that if change is to be effected, a mere increase in manpower is not enough. It is necessary to change the basis of the system and to radically change the system of delivery. Use of auxiliary personnel is fundamental, as is production of equipment at costs that can be readily absorbed. And finally, there is a need to develop specific disease control programs directed to specific population groups, to utilize clearly defined educational objectives for auxiliary personnel, and to develop specific guidelines for program implementation and evaluation.

ABOUT THE AUTHOR

Dr. Gillespie is the regional dental advisor in the Division of Family Health of the Pan American Health Organization. Prior to joining PAHO, Dr. Gillespie was chief of the Washington, D.C., dental care unit in the Division of Dental Health, U.S. Public Health Service. As such, he was early involved in dental care for Project Headstart. Before his government assignments, Dr. Gillespie was an assistant professor of dentistry at the University of Michigan.

Dr. Gillespie immigrated to North America from England, where he had received his B.D.S. degree in 1956. In 1963 he was awarded a D.D.S. degree from the University of Toronto, and he received an M.P.H. degree in 1964 from the University of Michigan.

In preparing Chapters 9 and 10, he was ably assisted by Drs. Ramon Covarey and Lorenzo Rivas of Venezuela and Dr. Patricio Yepes of Ecuador.

His present address is: Pan American Health Organization, 525 23rd Street, N.W., Washington, D.C. 20037.

✻ *Chapter 10*

Ecuador, A New Model

Dr. George M. Gillespie

Area: 273,724 square kilometers
Population: 6,730,000
Per Capita Gross National Product: $476 (ODC)
Life Expectancy: sixty years (ODC)

The experience in Venezuela led the government of Ecuador to enter into a similar dental care program emphasizing rural areas, where 68 percent of the population lives. Ecuador's program is operated by the Ministry of Health. In 1971, it was estimated that there were 1,000 dentists (and fourteen auxiliaries) in this relatively poor, small country, producing a distribution of one dentist per 3,000 urban population and one dentist to 60,000 in the rural areas. There were no preventive or community educational programs in dentistry, and rural dental care was extremely limited.

Then, in 1971, the Ministry of Health determined to change the pattern of delivery of health services. The first area selected for reform was that of administration, to consolidate the providers of health services into four easily defined and readily identified institutions: the Ministry of Health, Social Security, Armed Forces, and private practice. A Division of Dental Health was created with responsibility for planning, implementing, supervising, and evaluating national oral health programs. This division has two major components, a department of dental services and a department of research. Dental departments were also established in the twenty provinces of the country.

Unlike Venezuela, Ecuador's program is operated nationally by the Ministry of Health. It has shown the advantages that a centrally run program can provide in terms of national growth and continuity.

Preventive programs were introduced in 1972, with a law requiring fluoridation; some thirty-one cities, involving a population of 2,243,419 persons, are now fluoridating their water supplies. Self-application topical fluoride programs were started in 1975 and reached 53,000 children in 1976. Also in 1975, a fluoride mouthrinse program was begun with 63,000 children, which increased to 125,000 in 1976.

In connection with the revised administrative structure, all recent dental graduates were required to provide one year of service to the health authorities. They became the basic manpower for the rural program's new "dental brigades," which grew from seven in 1972 to twenty-two brigades and forty-two modules (106 dentists and 150 auxiliaries) in 1975. A brigade consists of two dentists and four locally recruited auxiliaries, who are taught basic functions of chairside assisting, dental prophylaxis, and prevention; all are employed by the Ministry of Health. Physical facilities are provided by the communities or, if not available, are built by the Ministry of Health. Dental care is provided with very simple equipment, which nonetheless includes both high speed and low speed air turbines, together with vacuum suction. PAHO/WHO collaborated in providing technical assistance to the Ministry in establishing these systems and in equipment design.

The original idea was that brigades would move from town to town. It soon became evident, however, that the concept of a rotating team produced little consistent community participation. The system was then modified to provide "modules" of one dentist and two auxiliaries working in a fixed location and remaining permanently on the site. By 1976, 159 modules were functioning involving 159 dentists and 349 auxiliaries. There were three remaining brigades. Some of the auxiliaries have been trained to do extractions and restorations, in addition to the chairside assisting and prophylaxis training normally given. Dental education and prevention is an integral part of the program, and particular attention is paid to school children. Productivity targets have been set, so that each team, or module, is expected to complete treatment on 1,100 patients a year.

In urban areas, especially in the health centers and hospitals, the same concepts were applied. New systems of practice were initiated, and an increase of 106 dentists and 94 auxiliaries was obtained. Fifty-four hospitals were reequipped.

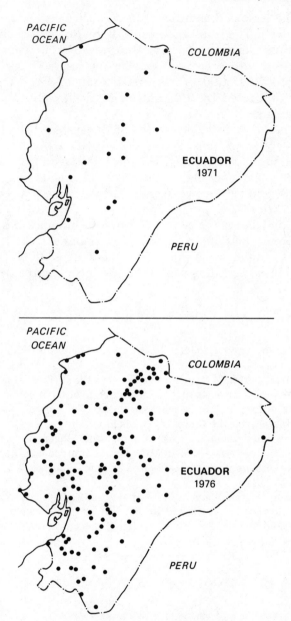

Figure 10–1. Geographic Distribution of Dental Health Services by the Ecuador Ministry of Public Health. *(The fivefold increase of clinics in five years (1971–1976) is dramatic proof of the high priority placed on dental care by the ministry.)*

Source: PAHO.

Clearly the lessons drawn from the Venezuela experience apply in Ecuador as well. The result has been a dramatic increase in the distribution of rural dental services and improved urban dental services. The population with access to dental care increased from 130,065 in June 1972 to 1,542,600 in the first quarter of 1977. On a budget completely supported by the Ministry of Health, that is a considerable achievement.

One of the most notable features of the system is that a fivefold increase in service has been accomplished with a budget that is little more than double what it was five years ago (see Figure 10—1). The estimated cost per completed treatment for a child is 25 sucres, or about $1.00, and preventive services are estimated at 1 cent for a thirty application, self-applied mouthrinse. The cost to set up the equipment and instruments for one of the modules has been estimated at around $4,000, investment in personnel at $34,000. Small health posts require an average investment of $2,000. Thus, in the rural situation in Ecuador, dental care can now be provided at a very realistic cost.

ABOUT THE AUTHOR

Dr. Gillespie is the regional dental advisor in the Division of Family Health of the Pan American Health Organization. Prior to joining PAHO, Dr. Gillespie was chief of the Washington, D.C., dental care unit in the Division of Dental Health, U.S. Public Health Service. As such, he was early involved in dental care for Project Headstart. Before his government assignments, Dr. Gillespie was an assistant professor of dentistry at the University of Michigan.

Dr. Gillespie immigrated to North America from England, where he had received his B.D.S. degree in 1956. In 1963 he was awarded a D.D.S. degree from the University of Toronto, and he received an M.P.H. degree in 1964 from the University of Michigan.

In preparing Chapters 9 and 10, he was ably assisted by Drs. Ramon Covarey and Lorenzo Rivas of Venezuela and Dr. Patricio Yepes of Ecuador.

His present address is: Pan American Health Organization, 525 23rd Street, N.W., Washington, D.C. 20037.

Chapter 11

Dental Care Delivery in the Republic of Cuba

Dr. Silvino Ruiz Miyares

Area: 111,111 square kilometers
Population: 9,137,000
Per Capita Income: $640 (ODC)
Life Expectancy: seventy years

After the triumph of the revolution, Cuban dentistry was in grave trouble. Out of the 2,000 dentists practicing in Cuba before the revolution, almost 800, as well as many dental students, left the country. During the early 1960s, due mainly to the drop in dental school enrollment, the number of dentists continued to decrease, while the population increased, making more precarious the ratio of dentists to inhabitants. There were no remaining dental auxiliaries in Cuba, and the only other providers left consisted of untrained "empiric" practitioners. Between 1966 and 1970, however, the situation began to turn around. The number of students increased, so that today Cuba graduates far more dentists than ever before. And just in time, too.

Seventeen years ago, we had about 30 percent illiteracy in Cuba. Now there is no illiteracy. The culture has accelerated and people are asking for a higher level of medical and dental care. Years ago, they asked only for extractions. Now they ask for restorative treatment, for prosthetic dentistry, and for orthodontic therapy for their children. When there is more development, people ask for more sophisticated things.

DENTAL MANPOWER

Today, there are 2,530 dentists in Cuba, which represents one dentist per 3,500 inhabitants. The country has two dental schools, now supervised by the Ministry of Public Health: an original one in Havana with 170 chairs, and a newer school (1967) in Santiago de Cuba with 70 chairs. Both follow a four year curriculum, with class sizes of 190 in Havana (about 60 percent female) and 50 in Santiago (about 90 percent female). Because entering classes in dentistry and medicine are allotted a fixed 20 percent of university enrollment (6.0 percent for dentistry and 14 percent for medicine), a huge increase is expected in 1978 related to increased university enrollment.

Dentists

Along with the medical students, the majority of dental students live free on campus. Like all Cuban students in high school and college, they are involved in a work-study program, initially serving as assistants to upper level students and later working in community and public health clinic programs. They are paid increasing amounts for this work, first through fourth year.

Following graduation, the new dentists will practice for three years in rural clinics, and some will then be chosen to move on into administration, to a more sophisticated setting, or into specialty training. In selecting new leaders, the ministry places great emphasis upon one's propensity for getting along well with patients and colleagues, as well as on professional ability. Young persons in positions of real responsibility are not at all unusual.

Specialists

In 1962, we began for the first time to train some dental specialists. More advanced specialty training—in orthodontics, prosthesis, periodontology, maxillofacial surgery, and public health management—dates from 1968. Cuba now has more than 185 specialists, with over 140 more undergoing training.

Specialty education is not limited to the two faculties of dentistry. Training centers are located in seven of fourteen provinces and are usually attached to larger public health clinics and staffed by specialists approved by the ministry. Orthodontists are being trained in Havana, Matanzas, Santa Clara, Camaguey, Holguin, and Santiago de Cuba. Prosthetists and periodontists are trained in Havana and Santiago de Cuba, while Camaguey also has facilities for prosthetic training. Public health management and basic research specialists are trained in Havana. Each provincial dental advisory group assesses the suitability of application for special training and determines its special needs in accordance with a national plan.[1]

Auxiliaries

The training of female dental clinical technicians (nurses) began in 1968, and 1,214 have graduated since 1970. There are 1,000 such nurses in active practice today, which means that, with the dentists, there is one operator for each 2,500 Cubans. A number of the dental nurses have been accepted into the dental schools and are now graduated as dentists. There is also considerable advancement of dental assistants into the dental nurse program.

Dental nurses are trained in restorative and preventive dentistry and radiographic techniques. It is no longer necessary that they learn to extract teeth. Their course has recently been extended from two to three years, beginning with grade nine; on completion, the women receive certification as clinical dental technicians while continuing with their general education.

The need for dental nurses is decreasing as more dentists are graduated, and classes have dropped from 200 nurses annually to 115. As students, they receive a small monthly stipend and live free of charge in dormitories on the top floors of the Havana school. Once they complete their training, they return to their home province to practice, alongside the dentists, in the many school and community clinics.

Other dental public health workers include:

1. 3,400 female dental assistants;
2. 130 technicians for the maintenance and repair of dental equipment; and
3. 685 dental prosthetic technicians who work in sixty-one laboratories around the nation.

DENTISTRY PROGRAMS

Dental care in Cuba is free, except for a small fee for prosthetic appliances.

The growth of treatment in dental care is even more dramatic than medical care. Between 1963 and 1974, dental consultations (appointments) increased over 800 percent, whereas medical appointments doubled during the same period (see Figure 11–1). As the Table 11–1 indicates, some headway has been made in improving the ratio of fillings to extractions, though we have not yet reached the optimum level.

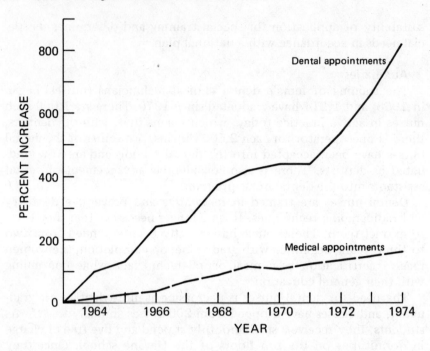

Figure 11–1. Dramatic Percentage Increase in Cuban Dental Appointments Reflects Ministry's Interest in Dental Care. *(Numerically, however, medical appointments far exceed dental ones.)*

Source: Cuba.

Clinics

Care is given in 133 dental clinics with more than five chairs each and in numerous smaller ones. Altogether, there are now more than 2,000 dental units (chairs) in Cuba. The fact that there are 1,500 more dentists and dental nurses than there are dental chairs reflects two factors. First, because of a shortage of foreign exchange, it has been very difficult for Cuba to bring in and maintain expensive dental equipment. Second, because most of the dental clinics operate twelve hours a day, from 8 A.M. to 9 P.M., including a half-day Saturday, it takes nearly a double shift of personnel to keep open. The long opening hours, to accommodate a working and student population, require more personnel.

Cuban dental clinics are found in polyclinics that provide primary health care of all sorts to a regional population. Polyclinic professional staff consists of family practice physicians, internists, obstetrician-gynecologists, pediatricians, dentists, and clinical dental

Table 11–1. Curative Services Rendered in Basic Programs. (Fourfold improvement in fillings to extraction rate is apparent.)

Year	Total Visits*	Fillings	Extractions	Fillings to Extraction Ratio
1965	1,556,000	776,000	1,541,000	0.5:1
1972	4,385,000	2,595,000	2,569,000	1.0:1
1973	5,330,000	3,401,000	2,731,000	1.2:1
1974	5,544,000	4,398,000	2,870,000	1.5:1
1975	6,969,000	4,861,000	2,730,000	1.7:1
1976 (est.)	7,200,000	5,655,000	2,759,000	2.0:1

*Includes specialist program visits.
Source: PAHO.

technicians. Large and small neighborhood clinics have been built in converted homes and other buildings. Dental equipment ranges from new units imported from Europe and Japan to prerevolutionary units that are gradually being phased out.

Many schools have their own dental clinic, while others are serviced in nearby neighborhood clinics or by mobile clinics. Every child, from the daycare centers through the university, may be examined and treated frequently, if necessary. Preventive programs have become part of a school's routine.

Many hospitals, including the small rural hospitals, have dental clinics, and specialty care is available in major hospitals and large clinics.

Specialized Dental Care

Table 11−2 offers graphic testimony to the rapid strides being taken in specialized dental care. As the table shows, there has been a 250 percent increase in endodontic treatment, a 167 percent increase in prosthetic services, and a 230 percent increase in orthodontic treatment. We have started an interceptive orthodontic service, involving the examination of children at their own schools in order to identify and treat developing problems early, thus preventing future malocclusions. In some provinces, all children seven to nine years old have been examined, and removable orthodontic appliances and head gears are a common sight. This treatment is rendered mostly by postdoctoral students being trained in specialty clinics.

There are also special dental programs for target groups of the population, particularly pregnant women and daycare and primary school children. These groups are supposed to receive 9 percent, 3 percent, and 25 percent, respectively, of the basic care time available. All the programs include several aspects of health education.

• Every pregnant woman is asked by her physician to go to the dentist. Over 37,000 received services in the dental clinics in 1976, and 26,500—or about 25 percent of the target group—had a treatment plan completed in 1977.
• Children three to five years old receive dental care through clinics associated with the daycare centers they attend.
• Neighborhood dental clinics devote 20−25 percent of their time to the care of primary school children. About one in nine children from the ages of six to twelve received care in 1976. Over 780,000 fillings were made, with a ratio of four fillings per extraction of either deciduous or permanent teeth.

Table 11–2. Specialized Dentistry in Cuba. *(Dramatic increase in programs aimed at retention of dentition is the goal.)*

	1973	1975	1976	Percent of Increase
Endodontics (treatment to population ratio)	1:453	1:220	1:179	250
Prosthetics (treatment to population ratio over age fifteen)	1:90	1:63	1:54	167
Orthodontics (treatment to population ratio for ages six to fourteen	1:1,456	1:772	1:631	230

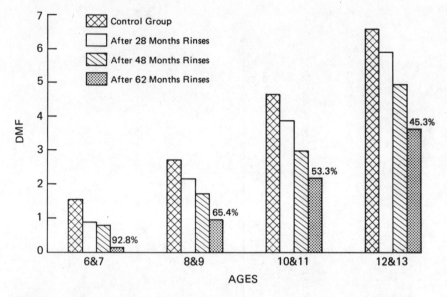

Figure 11–2.   Reduction in DMF rate in Cuba Credited in Part to Fluoride Rinse Program. *(Dramatic drop after five years ranges from 45 percent to 93 percent according to age.)*

Source: Cuba.

A preventive program for this age group was launched in 1969. It consists of mouthwashes with an 0.2 percent sodium fluoride solution every fifteen days[2] for school children and the application of fluoride lacquer twice a year to daycare children[3] and others who attend schools far from urban areas. Over 900,000 children receive preventive care by dental assistants from the Ministry of Public Health, with the cooperation of volunteer members of the sanitary brigades of the Federation of Cuban Women; the latter have received a course in basic health measures.[4]

This preventive care program has been very successful and extraordinarily inexpensive. Figure 11–2 shows the decrease of caries incidence due to the sodium fluoride mouthwashes.[5]

PERSPECTIVES, 1976–1980

Expansion of the Dental Delivery System

At present, a "sectorized" system for dental care is being implemented to cover all 14 provinces of Cuba. Under this system, each dentist, helped by clinical dental nurses and assistants, will provide care to a population sector having an average of 3,000 inhabitants.

Patients requiring the attention of a specialist will be referred to the secondary level of dental care.[6]

In order to achieve more complete coverage, several new dental clinics with twenty chairs are under construction, as are laboratories for twenty prosthetic technicians. These clinics will be located in the principal cities of the country. By 1980, more than one hundred additional polyclinics and hospitals will be built; each will include dental services having five to fourteen chairs.

During this period, over 1,000 dentists will be graduated, and we will continue the training of specialists as well as auxiliary personnel.

Fluoridation

The small community of La Salud (6,500 inhabitants) has had artificially fluoridated water since 1972. During 1977 and the first half of 1978, the fluoridation of eight more communities will begin, covering a total population of 174,000.[7] This will be a starting point for enlarging the fluoridation of the drinking water system. (Bottled drinking water already has one part per million of fluoride.)

Dental Care in High Schools

The next major target group to receive systematic treatment will be adolescents. There are already over one hundred dental units attached to high schools in the countryside. This year another 150 simplified units in three unit modules are being developed under a cooperative program with UNICEF and the Pan American Health Organization. With these modules, we expect to spend about three months at any one high school (average 500 students) for primary treatment—restorative, endodontics, exodontics, and prophylaxis. We will then transfer the module to another school. Thus, with each three units, we can finish treatment of at least three schools in one school year. Once the initial care cycle is finished, we will begin the maintenance stage, along with treatment of entering students. In this way, we expect to reach no less than 400,000 high school students and those from other schools in the countryside by 1980.

CONCLUSIONS

These are some aspects of the dental programs currently functioning in Cuba. D.W. Lewis, from the University of Toronto, who visited our country in May 1977 to study our dental care delivery system, has observed:

> It can be said with confidence that the present dental system of Cuba demonstrates how a society can develop, in a relatively short number of years,

a good dental care system through careful integrative planning, allocation of sufficient funds, and dedication to the social policy that, since dental health is important, dental care should be available to all.[8]

With the personnel and equipment in prospect for 1980—some of it already functioning—we expect to improve the quality and to increase the amount of the services provided to our population, as it is the one and only objective of our dental profession.

NOTES

1. S. Ruiz Miyares, El Desarrollo de la Estomatología en Cuba, conferencia durante el Taller de Atencion Odontologica a la Comunidad, La Habana, OPS/OMS, September 6—14, 1976,

2. H. Berggren, Fluoruros de Uso Topico (incluyendo los dentifricos), *Int. Dent. Journal* 17, No. 1 (1967): 44—46; P. Torell and F. Erickson, The Value in Caries Prevention of Methods for Applying Fluroides Topically to the Teeth, *Int. Dent. Journal* 17 (September 1967): 564; P. Torell and F. Erickson, Two Years Clinical Test with Different Methods of Local Caries Prevention Fluorine Applications in Swedish School-Children, *Acta Odont. Scand.* 23 (1967): 287; and B.V. Miguel Martín, Programa Incremental de Atencion Estomatologica a Escolares de Primaria en la Provincia de Las Villas, Cuba, 1970—1975 (Trabajo presentado en el Congreso Odontologico Internacional en Lima, Peru, Dic. 1975).

3. G. Heuser and H.F.M. Schmidt, Topical Application of Fluorine Lacquer, *Stoma* 2 (1970): 91.

4. F. Soto Padrón and H.J. Maiwald, Analisis de los Resulta dos de las Aplicaciones Topicas de Fluoruros a Grupos de Población en Cuba, *Rev. Cub. Estom.* 10 (1973): 173.

5. F. Soto, W. Kunzel, and S. Ruiz Miyares, Resultados obtenidos por èl Empleo de Soluciones de Fluoruro de Sodio al 0.2% en Enjuagatorios Realizados Masivamente (despues de 62 meses de control), *Rev. Cub. Estom.* 13 (1976); 1—5.

6. Ministerio de Salud Publica de Cuba, *Fundamentación para un Nuevo Enfoque de la Medicina en la Comunidad* (Havana, 1975); and Ministerio de Salud Pública de Cuba, *Proyecto de Reglamento de Policlínico Integral*, En proceso de analisis (Havana, 1977).

7. CUBA-UNICEF-OPS/OMS, *Programa Integral Estomatologico Dirigido a los Grupos Escolares de la Republica de Cuba* (Havana, 1975).

8. D.W. Lewis, *The Dental Care System of Cuba, 1977*, Research Report, The Faculty of Dentistry (Toronto: University of Toronto, June 1977).

ABOUT THE AUTHOR

Dr. Silvino Miyares is the national chief of stomatology in the Ministry of Public Health in Cuba. Prior to becoming the nation's chief dental officer, he conducted a private practice from 1953 until 1962. Following the revolution in 1959, Dr. Miyares served in various capacities in the ministry. He also served on the faculties of the Schools of Dentistry at University of Havana and at Oriente University in Santiago de Cuba. In 1968 and 1969, Dr. Miyares was a teacher of operative dentistry at the Havana school for dental nurses.

Born in Las Villas province, he received his B.S. degree in 1948 and was graduated with a D.D.S. from the University of Havana in 1953.

His present address is: Jéfe de Estomatologia, Ministerio de Salud Publica, Habana, Cuba.

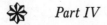 *Part IV*

The European Experience

Surely there is a lesson to be learned from the multitude of dental care delivery systems extant in Europe. Each nation appears to have gone its own way in solving its dental care problems. This diversity of approach ranges from total socialism to staunch free enterprise.

Although the organizers of this conference would have preferred to present a wider array of European nations, the countries here represented are quite selective of movements presently underway. Programs of some of the missing nations are discussed in Part VII, Audience Participation.

Chapter 12

Dental Care Delivery in the United Kingdom (England and Wales)

Michael A. Lennon

Area: 244,000 square kilometers (all U.K.)
Population: 49,200,000 (56,100,000 all U.K.)
Per Capita Gross National Product: $3,590 (all U.K.)
Life Expectancy: seventy-two years (all U.K.)

In the United Kingdom, dental care is provided through three distinct systems (see Table 12—1): the School Dental Service, providing inspection and treatment for school children and employing about 10 percent of all dentists on a salaried basis; the General Dental Service, employing about 80 percent of all dentists and providing treatment on demand to the general population, including children; and the Hospital Dental Service, providing specialist orthodontic and oral-surgical advice and treatment to patients referred from the other

Table 12—1. Dental Systems in the United Kingdom.

Service	Patients	Dentists (1974)	
		Number	Percent
School dental service	Children	1,585*	10
General dental service	Adults and Children	12,500	80
Hospital dental service	Referred Patients	832*	5
Other	—	—	5

*Full-time Equivalent.

two services and employing about 5.0 percent of all dentists, again on a salaried basis. Data on private practice are not available; the purely private practitioner is rare, but the average general dental practitioner seems to spend about 10 percent of his time on private patients.

Details of the salaried school and hospital services have been published elsewhere[1] and these references, together with basic demographic and manpower data, appear as an appendix to this chapter. Here I shall concentrate on the General Dental Service—first, because this is by far the largest of the three branches of our dental services (indeed, it is treating three times as many children as the School Dental Service) and, second, because its system of cost control is unique and, therefore, of particular interest. We are talking about a service that has been in existence for almost thirty years, that involves almost 13,000 dentists, and that, in 1975, provided over twenty-eight million courses of treatment at a cost of over $330 million to a population of almost fifty million.[2] Thus, it is a relatively large service with a long history and a complex and evolving organization. (Scotland and Northern Ireland have parallel delivery systems, but this chapter concerns only those for England and Wales.)

The following four sections (1) describe the situation that existed before 1948, when the service was first established, and describe the early aims and organization of the service; (2) discuss the experiences of the service during its first ten years, highlighting some of the problems, particularly in the area of cost control; (3) detail the reorganization of the systems of remunerating dentists and of cost control that came about in an attempt to solve some of these problems; and finally, (4) evaluate the performance of the service over the past fifteen years and in particular consider its efficiency, its adequacy, and its effectiveness.

ORIGIN OF THE GENERAL DENTAL SERVICE

Before 1948, only the most rudimentary dental services were available to the general population, and less than 10 percent of the population made a dental visit in any one year. The dental health of the population was appalling. In addition—indeed, because of this low demand–high need situation—the dental profession itself was in a poor state; recruitment was low, and the profession was reducing in size; 50 percent of all dentists were over fifty years of age, and these older dentists were retiring more quickly than new dentists were being trained.[3]

There appeared to be two reasons for this state of affairs: first, the poor attitude of the population toward dental health and dental treatment and, second, their inability to afford the cost of treatment. While the former attitude was considered the more fundamental problem, the cost of treatment was more amenable to change. Reducing the cost of treatment, it was thought, would stimulate demand, and as demand increased, attitudes would begin to improve, as would recruitment to the profession.

Thus, there were two aims when the service was instituted in 1948:

1. To increase the demand for dental treatment from the general population, and
2. To stimulate recruitment to the dental profession.

To better understand the growth and functioning of the service, one must review the regulations governing its operation. Regulations allow any registered dentist to contract to provide dental treatment under the service. The dentist remains a completely independent practitioner. He sets up his practice in any part of the country he wishes, he owns the practice, he hires and fires his own staff, and he treats as many or as few patients as he wishes. He simply places his name on the list of dentists maintained in any one of the ninety-eight administrative areas in England and Wales, and he is then, in effect, a National Health Service dentist.

A patient wishing treatment under the service approaches a dentist; the dentist in his turn may accept or reject the patient, but, having accepted the patient, contracts to provide all treatment necessary for dental fitness that the patient is prepared to accept. (Dental fitness is defined as that level of dental health necessary to protect general health, a rather vague and elastic definition.) Once the course of treatment is successfully completed, the dentist's obligation to that patient ceases; he has no responsibility to recall him or to see him again for maintenance care. In this respect, the dental service is quite unlike the medical services, where patients are registered with their doctors, and the doctor has an ongoing responsibility to his list of patients.

The patient, and there are about twenty million per year, seeks treatment from one of the 13,000 dentists who are on contract with one of the ninety-eight Area Health Authorities (Family Practitioner Committees). When the course of treatment is complete, the dentist sends a claim form for his fee to a central administrative organization, the Dental Estimates Board, which checks and sanctions the fee and informs the Area Health Authority (Family Practitioner Committee). At the end of each month, the latter authority pays the dentist his accumulated fees for that month (see Figure 12—1). The fee schedule is based on a fee for item of service, with the exception of certain more complex treatments, such as orthodontics, where an appropriate fee is negotiated for each course of treatment before it is carried out.

THE EARLY YEARS, 1948—1958

The fee for item of service system imposed considerable strains on the service in the first ten years. Within a few months of its inception, the service was almost overwhelmed by a demand for treatment, more than twice the predicted rate.[4] This demand was essentially from the adult and elderly population, for the extraction of septic teeth and their replacement with dentures. In addition, dentists were working at a greater rate and for longer hours than previously. As a result, the cost of the dental service was far greater than had been expected—over 10 percent of the total National Health Service bill. Of every £10 spent on the National Health Service in 1948, £1 went to dentistry and a large proportion of that on dentures. The government panicked. Cuts in the fee schedule were introduced within nine months, in February 1949, again in June 1949, and still further in May 1950. In May 1951, patient surcharges were introduced on dentures, and in June 1952, this surcharge was extended to all courses of treatment for adults over twenty-one years of age.

These changes in fees and regulations were introduced by the government quite unilaterally; there was no consultation with the British Dental Association. As a result, relationships between, on the

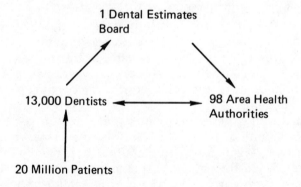

Figure 12—1. Administrative Organization for the General Dental Service.

one hand, physicians and dentists (because physicians were having similar problems) and, on the other hand, the government became very poor. Physicians and dentists came to believe that their pay was subject to the whim of the minister of health and that the government was in some way using physician and dentist pay to regulate, or at least to influence, pay in other professions and in industry. Whether this was true or not does not matter; what did matter was that physicians and dentists thought it was true. Clearly, the harmonious administration of a service becomes very difficult under such circumstances.

REORGANIZATION OF REMUNERATION AND COST CONTROL

As a result of this deep disquiet, a royal commission was appointed to investigate physician and dentist pay. The commission was set the task of finding some way of regulating remuneration and costs acceptable to the professions, to the government, and to the public. Its recommendations[5] with regard to dentistry were implemented in 1961 and have formed the basis for financing the service ever since.

Although we have retained the fee per item of service system, the whole basis for the calculation of the fee schedule has been altered. Up to 1958, the fee schedule itself formed the basis for negotiation, which, as we have already noted, led to a cost explosion. After 1961, the whole system was flipped over on its head, and the dentist's net earnings became the negotiable factor. Once a decision had been agreed between government and the profession on what the average dentist should net, and given adequate data on dentist productivity and practice expenses, then the calculation of the necessary gross income and the appropriate fee schedule could, as it were, be passed over to the statisticians.

What actually happens is that there are two committees, the Review Body and the Dental Rates Study Group. The role of the Review Body is to recommend what the average dentist should net; the Dental Rates Study Group then calculates the fee schedule.

The Review Body is independent of the government and professions; it is made up of eminent men and women in public life—leaders in industry and the unions, professors of economics, and the like—who, after receiving evidence from all sides, exercise their judgment as to what the dentist should reasonably earn, taking into account movements in salaries in industry, other professions, and so on. Their advice is given directly to the prime minister, who is under strong pressure to accept it.

The second committee is the Dental Rates Study Group, which is made up of equal numbers of representatives from the government (Department of Health and Social Security) and from the British Dental Association, with an independent chairman. They carry out what is, in effect, a complicated statistical exercise to calculate, first, what additional money the average dentist must earn over the Review Body's recommended net income in order to cover his practice expenses and, second, the appropriate fee schedule, so that the average dentist working at the average speed will earn the recommended average net income.

By this device, a very difficult situation was defused. The profession and the government no longer met over a table to haggle over fees. The government, for its part, was no longer able to cut fees unilaterally, and yet the level of fees charged was not left simply to be determined by dentists and market forces. The system, which is still evolving, has worked reasonably well, although our recent rapid inflation has caused problems in the prediction of practice expenses. The system has undoubtedly been a major factor in promoting the overall efficiency of our delivery system.

1961–1976: AN EVALUATION

In this section, I shall follow the recommendations of the World Health Organization's 1972 report[6] on the evaluation of dental services and consider efficiency, adequacy, and effectiveness.

Efficiency may be defined as the cost, or perhaps the relative cost, of a unit output. In our system of remuneration, there is a built-in stimulus to efficiency. Because the fee schedule is rigidly fixed from year to year, the dentist can only increase his income by increasing his output or by reducing his overhead expenses. One manifestation of this is the movement toward economies of scale. In 1956, 59 percent of general dental practitioners were in solo practice. The most recent survey (Figure 12–2) suggests that the equivalent figure in 1975 was only 22 percent, with 49 percent of practitioners in the service in group practices of three dentists or more.[7]

There is little doubt that the British public and the government receive their dental care at relatively low cost. In 1972, though the figures are a little out of date now, we compared dentist total earnings and the cost of a single item of treatment—full upper and lower dentures—in each of six countries.[8] To standardize these figures, both the dentist's average weekly income and the cost of the dentures were expressed as a proportion of the average industrial worker's wage in each of the countries. As Table 12–2 shows, by and

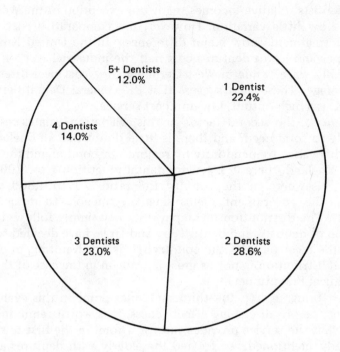

Figure 12—2. Practice Size in the General Dental Service, 1975.

Source: British Dental Association.

Table 12—2. International Comparative Costs and Income, 1968—1969.
(Relative cost of dentures in the U.K. is one-third to one-sixth the cost elsewhere. Outside of West Germany there was little variation in dentist's relative income.)

	Dentist's Weekly Income	Cost of Full Dentures
	Average Industrial Worker's Weekly Wage	Average Industrial Worker's Weekly Wage
U.K.	2.8	0.5
Australia	3.0	1.4
New Zealand	3.6	1.4
Canada	3.5	2.0
U.S.A.	3.2	2.0
West Germany	7.4	3.1

large, dentists' relative incomes, with the exception of the West Germans, show little variation. However, the comparative costs of an item of treatment show major differences. In the United Kingdom, full upper and lower dentures cost half the industrial worker's average weekly wage, while in West Germany they cost over three times that average. These data suggest that the General Dental Service in the U.K. is a high output, low unit cost service.

Adequacy, the second factor in this evaluation, relates resources available to total need, and there is little doubt that in England and Wales this varies tremendously by region.[9] In London and the southeast of England, there is 1 general dental practitioner to 3,000 population; elsewhere in the country the ratio is 1 to 4,800, and at present, the government seems singularly unable to do anything about it. The distribution of taxpayer money simply follows the distribution of dentists, and dentists, by and large, have decided to practice in the nicer parts of the country. (It is worth noting, in passing, that maldistribution is not as great a problem in the case of the General Medical Practitioners.)

Which brings me to the third and final point in this evaluation. However, before discussing effectiveness, it is worth reminding ourselves what the service provides and for whom. In the first few years, as already mentioned, we treated the elderly with dentures and extractions. Today, we are providing restorative dentistry for the young; about half of all courses of treatment are for people under twenty-one years of age. If we look at a breakdown of current costs (Figure 12–3), we see that 17 percent of total expenditures is on examination and x-rays, 32 percent on simple restorations, and a further 19 percent on acrylic dentures. Negligible amounts of money are spent on preventive advice and treatment and negligible amounts on periodontal care. In other words, we spend almost all our resources on the treatment of dental disease. How effective is this service?

Effectiveness may be defined as the extent to which a service achieves its aims, and its evaluation requires that such aims have been clearly stated from the outset. I already mentioned two aims: increased demand for treatment and improved recruitment to the dental profession. Both of these have been reasonably achieved. The amount of treatment has trebled from 177 courses of treatment per 1,000 population to the present 552 courses per 1,000, while the number of dental students has increased by over 50 percent in the last twenty years. But it would not seem unreasonable to assume that the service had aims other than simply increasing the amount of dental treatment carried out. One might assume, for example, that some

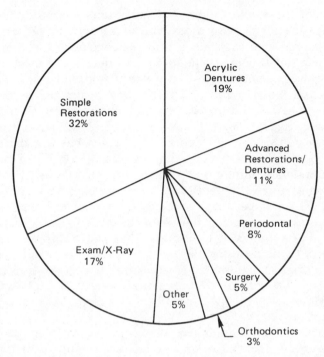

Figure 12–3. Costs as a Percentage of the Total Costs in the General Dental Service.

Source: British Dental Association.

improvement in dental health was envisaged—say, a reduction in dental sepsis or a reduction in tooth loss.

There is little doubt, as the 1968 National Survey of Adult Dental Health[10] showed, that gross oral sepsis is a thing of the past. Even those who make least use of the service, the irregular attenders, show very little evidence of gross dental disease. The average adult irregular attender, aged sixteen years and over, has less than one tooth requiring extraction and 2.4 teeth requiring filling, and this need shows little variation by age, sex, social class, or geographical region. When we bear in mind that, in 1968, 75 percent of even the irregular attenders had made a dental visit in the previous five years, it is not unreasonable to conclude that the service is accessible and provides a very basic level of dental health to the total population.

Our second assumed objective was a reduction in tooth loss. Here, again, there are problems in deciding the most appropriate forms of data, but some insight may be gained by comparing the state of dental health of those who choose to make optimum use of the service—the regular attenders—with those who make only limited use,[11] even though one must be cautious in drawing conclusions from comparisons of such self-selected populations. The data, again from the 1968 national sruvey, demonstrate that the regular attender, in spite of his yearly dental examination and restorative treatment, is still losing teeth; he loses them more slowly than the irregular attender but, nevertheless, he still loses them (Table 12—3). A more recent national survey, this time in Scotland[12] (which has the same dental services, but with a separate administration), concluded that "we have a considerable number of people with high levels of tooth loss who chose to go to the dentist for a regular check up. . . . It would appear that, for these people, regular attendance has not been altogether successful in saving their natural teeth." Thus, Holloway[13] formulated the tentative hypothesis that the restorative approach to dentistry (which is what the General Dental Service at its best provides) is palliative rather than therapeutic; it postpones rather than prevents the breakdown of the natural dentition. Holloway cited similar evidence from New Zealand and the United States to support his contention.

In conclusion and summary, therefore, we have in the United Kingdom considerable experience in delivering dental care in an organized way to a large population. After initial serious problems in controlling costs, we have now developed a system that promotes high output at low cost. The service has ensured a basic minimum level of dental health to the entire population.

On the debit side, first, the service is still poorly distributed geographically, and there is at present considerable public debate on this issue. Second, there is growing concern, at least among our dental epidemiologists,[14] that the main aim of our service, the provision of regular dental examination and restorative treatment, may not by itself guarantee the maintenance of the natural dentition.

Table 12—3. Tooth Loss in the U.K. in Regular and Irregular Attenders, by Age, 1968.

Age	Missing Teeth	
	Regular	Irregular
16–34	5.5	7.8
35+	10.4	15.5

APPENDIX

DEMOGRAPHY, HEALTH EXPENDITURE, AND MANPOWER

Demography
The United Kingdom combines in a political union England, Wales, Scotland, and Northern Ireland. For the purposes of dental health administration, England and Wales may be considered as a single unit, with separate administrations for Scotland and Northern Ireland. This chapter deals with England and Wales only, unless otherwise stated.

Health Expenditures
The Gross Domestic Product in 1975 was £94 billion, of which £7 billion (7.4 percent) was spent on health and welfare. Of this £7 billion, a little less than 5 percent was spent on dental services.

Manpower
All dentists, dental hygienists, and dental auxiliaries wishing to practice are required to register annually with the General Dental Council. The names of registered dentists and ancillary workers are published annually for the whole of the United Kingdom.

Number on Register as of January 1, 1977:

Dentists   19,956

Approximately 2,000 of these dentists are sixty-five years old or more.

Dental Hygienists   901

The dental hygienist can work in the hospital service, the school service, or in the general dental service. More are needed, and the government is taking steps to increase the number in training.

New Cross Dental Auxiliaries   462

The New Cross dental auxiliary can work only in the school dental service, carrying out simple restorative dentistry. The recent report[15] on child health services in England recommends that two new schools for New Cross dental auxiliaries be built, but the wisdom of increasing the number of these ancillary workers is still a matter of some controversy. The arguments center on economics. The dentist in the United Kingdom is already providing efficient and low cost care. A dental auxiliary has about the same operating expenses as the dentist, so the difference between the cost of employing an auxiliary and employing a dentist is not as dramatic as it might at first appear. Thus, the British Dental Association has taken the position that the New Cross dental scheme requires further evaluation before expansion should be considered.

Income Levels (approximate averages, mid-1976)

Dentists

General Dental Service
(average net income)   £8,000 per annum

School Dental Service
Dental Officer (salary)   £4,500–£6,600 per annum

Hospital Dental Service
Consultant Oral Surgeon (salary)   £7,500–£10,700 per annum

Dental Hygienist

Hospital and School
Dental Services (salary)   £2,500–£3,200 per annum

General Dental Service   Negotiable with practice
                                      principal—probably a little
                                      higher than above

Dental Auxiliary

Hospital and School
Dental Services (salary)   £2,500–£3,700 per annum

*Average Industrial Worker's
Earnings*   £4,000 per annum

NOTES

1. G.L. Howe, Dentistry in the National Health Service of the United Kingdom: Some thoughts on the Hospital Dental Service, *International Dental Journal* 25 (1975): 120–25; and G.B. Winter, A paedodontist's view of child dental care in the United Kingdom, *International Dental Journal* 25 (1975): 126–31.

2. Department of Health and Social Security, Dental Estimates Board Annual Report for 1975 (London: 1976).

3. Teviot Report, Interdepartmental committee on dentistry—Interim Report (London: H.M.S.O., 1944).

4. N.D. Richards, Social Sciences and Dentistry, eds. N.D. Richards and L.K. Cohen (The Hague: Sijthoff, 1971), p. 209.

5. *Royal Commission on Doctors and Dentists Remuneration* (London: H.M.S.O., 1960).

6. World Health Organization, *Planning and Evaluating Dental Health Services* (Copenhagen: WHO, 1972).

7. British Dental Association, Economies of scale in dental practice. *British Dental Journal* 141 (1976): 191–92.

8. British Dental Association, Seventh Memorandum to the Review Body, *British Dental Journal* 133 (1972): 71–73.

9. M.A. Lennon, An evaluation of the adequacy of the General Dental Service, *British Dental Journal* 141 (1976): 223–25.

10. P.G. Gray, J.E. Todd, G.L. Slack, and J.S. Bulman, *Adult Dental Health in England and Wales in 1968* (London: H.M.S.O., 1970).

11. P.J. Holloway, The success of restorative dentistry? *International Dental Journal* 25 (1975): 26–30.

12. J.E. Todd, and A. Whitworth, *Adult dental health in Scotland, 1972* (London: H.M.S.O., 1974).

13. Holloway.

14. D. Jackson, J.J. Murray, and C.G. Fairpo, Regular dental care in dentate persons, *British Dental Journal* 135 (1973): 59–63; A. Sheiham, An evaluation of the success of dental care in the United Kingdom, *British Dental Journal* 135 (1973): 271–79; Holloway; and Todd and Whitworth.

15. *The report of the Committee on Child Health Services* (London: H.M.-S.O., 1976); Diana M. Scarrott, The economic case for delegation in dentistry, *British Dental Journal* 134 (1973): 23–24; and British Dental Association, The developing role of dental ancillary personnel, *British Dental Journal* 141 (1976): 51–53.

ABOUT THE AUTHOR

Michael Lennon is a lecturer in community dentistry in the Department of Preventive Dentistry at the University Dental Hospital of Manchester in England. As such he has become an astute observer of the British dental scene, serving as secretary of the British Association for the Study of Community Dentistry.

Mr. Lennon received his dental degree (B.D.S.) from the University of Liverpool in 1966. Since that time he has received a D.P.D. degree from the University of Dundee in Scotland and an M.D.S. degree from the University of Manchester. He is also a fellow of the Royal College of Surgeons of Edinburgh.

His present address is: Department of Preventive Dentistry, University Dental Hospital of Manchester, Manchester, United Kingdom.

Chapter 13

Dental Care Delivery in Czechoslovakia

Dr. Jarmil Kostlán

Area: 132,000 square kilometers
Population: 15,000,000
Per Capita Gross National Product: $3,590
    (1974 estimated; ODC)
Life Expectancy: seventy years

Dental service in Czechoslovakia is governmental. It is fully socialized, being developed in accordance with state economic plans, financed from the state budget, and delivered free of charge to consumers by salaried dentists through a network of basic and specialized dental health centers. This system, which was introduced in 1951, does not represent as radical a change for Czechoslovaks as it might have for citizens of some other countries. Private dental insurance existed as far back as 1900, when Czechoslovakia was still part of the Austro-Hungarian Empire; and in 1948, the government established a state run National Dental Health Insurance, under which most dental services were transferred to public polyclinics.

The amount spent for dental health service cannot be ascertained precisely, because many dental services and facilities are closely integrated with general health services. It is clear, however, that the total is quite large. In 1975, every third person touched by the outpatient health services was a dental patient.

DENTAL MANPOWER

By 1975, Czechoslovakia had 6,434 dentists, for a dentist to population ratio of 1:2,500. More than 60 percent of the dentists are

111

women. Nine out of ten dentists work for a dental health service that falls under the Ministry of Health; the remainder work in special dental services attached to the armed forces and railroads or teach or undertake research in one of our ten dental schools.

Private dental practice has not been abandoned. Dentists who do not have enough service years to qualify for a pension, for example, are permitted to open private surgeries. But private dentistry accounts for less than 1 percent of the total. After the national dental service was introduced, we found that patients' interest in private dentistry dropped surprisingly rapidly—in two or three years, in fact—though some patients still grumble that the dentist's interest in them is not as warm and close as it might be if he had his own practice.

Stomatologists—dentists with a university education—are produced by the ten stomatological university clinics affiliated with medical schools. Before 1952, the old Austrian pattern was followed: a stomatologist had to finish his medical studies before taking a two year postgraduate course in stomatology. Today, only an aging minority of dentists were trained this way. The process was too long and expensive and was attracting too few students, so the system was abandoned in favor of a five year undergraduate curriculum. This curriculum comprises nearly all the biological and medical subjects characteristic of medical education, but it emphasizes dental subjects in clinical training. In addition to their regular training, students spend one semester in the field working at dental health centers. Graduates obtain the title of M.D., but they are restricted by regulation of the Ministry of Health to work in the dental field.

After graduation, dentists enter the governmental dental health service network. The young dentist can choose the locality where he will practice from among the vacant posts that are advertised at the dean's office in the dental school. After three years, he must undergo a so-called attestation examination in order to prove that he has mastered the full scope of dental prevention and treatment required in general practice. His salary then rises, and he can decide whether he wants to continue working as a general practitioner, move into dental service administration, or specialize.

Three year courses are available in one of four dental specialities—maxillofacial surgery, children's dentistry, orthodontics, and periodontology. Specialization in prosthetic dentistry has now been abolished. All dentists are supposed to take part in continuous postgraduate education, which is organized by special postgraduate training institutes. Both undergraduate and postgraduate training are free of charge.

A peculiar feature of our dental service is that about 19 percent of our dentists are former dental technicians who were authorized, on the basis of a special examination, to treat dental patients. These days, this now aging category is successfully being replaced by university-trained stomatologists. It was first introduced in the 1920s, and then again for a few years after World War II, when closure of the universities and political and religious persecution under the German occupation had resulted in a severe shortage of dental manpower. Some districts had only one dentist for 30,000 people, and one-third of the districts were without any dentist at all. Obviously, the government had to do something forceful to help people keep dental service at a reasonable level.

There are about 12,000 dental auxiliaries in Czechoslovakia. Some 6,500 function as dental assistants and the remainder as dental technicians. In the former category, many dental departments—especially those for oral surgery and children's dentistry—employ medical nurses and encourage their chairside assistants to achieve professional education comparable to that of a trained nurse. Dentists seem to feel that having a well-educated medical nurse enhances their own status; also, the state health administration seems to find it easier to handle all the different auxiliaries as if they were interchangeable. But if the auxiliary lacks dental training, she must be retrained. This strikes me as poor economics.

Both the dental assistants and the technicians graduate from a four year special school that, like the dental schools, is free. Their final examination fulfills the condition for university entrance. Postgraduate training is available for auxiliaries wishing to specialize.

Auxiliaries similar to dental hygienists are seldom used; only a few hundred dental assistants or nurses have taken special theoretical and practical training courses to become hygienists. Dental therapists and New Zealand type school dental nurses are not used at all. Auxiliaries have their own professional organization and may become members of the stomatological association.

BASIC FEATURES OF THE CZECH DENTAL HEALTH SERVICE

Planning

The national Ministry of Health is concerned with overall planning and evaluation of the dental service and with long-term analysis of its needs and working conditions. Planning takes place in several time frames. Long-term plans look forward several decades to consider general trends and conditions necessary for the service's development. Medium-term plans, usually prepared for five year periods, deal with the strategy of curative and preventive services. Finally, short-term plans are prepared for every calendar year to govern operations. These plans are prepared very thoroughly, and—once agreed upon and officially accepted—are binding for all.

National Priorities

A right to be healthy and to have access to health service is granted to every citizen by the state constitution. Health care, including all sorts of dental service, is in principle free of charge, though nominal charges are levied for gold restorations and for construction of fixed prosthetic appliances.

The service's aim is to treat the adult population according to their demand for service and to provide treatment to preferential population groups, especially children, on the basis of need. Top priority is given to preventing tooth loss. We try to deliver as many fillings as possible, and we try to start as early in childhood as possible. We emphasize to our dentists that a simple filling is much better than a filling that has to be preceded by pulpal treatment, and extraction is, of course, worse than filling after pulpal treatment. Our data show that simple fillings made in time are important for the preservation of natural dentition.

Delivery of Services

The operation of the service is delegated to lower echelons of administration, with coordination secured by chief stomatologists at each administrative level. The chief stomatologist of the Ministry of Health and his regional and district counterparts are responsible for the realization of the dental health services concept, for the quality of its work, and for the continuous education of its manpower.

Territorialization of the Service Network. The whole country is divided into so-called health areas, with each elementary health area comprising an average of about 3,500 inhabitants. The primary health service team working in each area consists of a general practitioner and his nurse, a stomatologist and his dental assistant, and a part-time pediatrician and gynecologist with their medical auxiliaries. This system enables the dentist to take advantage of the general health services to organize care for adults and adolescents; for example, when these groups come to the health center for immunization and the like, they can also be sent to the dental center for screening.

There are also dental clinics in the factories, in big offices, and in other workplaces.

Special dental health service is available at both the district and regional levels. (A district usually comprises about 100,000 inhabitants and a region between half and one and a half million inhabitants.) In the district towns, there are one or more dental polyclinics, employing both general dental practitioners to treat local patients and specialists to deal with difficult cases sent there from the whole district. These polyclinics have at least one specialist in dental surgery and, frequently, specialists in pedodontics and orthodontics. In well-staffed polyclinics, there are also departments for prosthodontics and periodontology. Specialists also undertake to train general dental practitioners in their specialty.

In each regional town, there is a regional dental health center with an inpatient and an outpatient department. Patients needing treatment are sent at the expense of the dental health service administration; even travel expenses are reimbursed. Full sets of dental specialists work in the outpatient departments. There are twenty-eight inpatient departments, but some of them are small and uneconomic; the trend in thinking, at least in the state health administration, is to cut down the number of these hospital departments and to upgrade outpatient services instead.

This system secures a very even availability and accessibility of both basic and special services over the whole country. On the other hand, it limits the patient's choice of dentists. However, the patient can choose either the dentist working near his home or near the place where he works; and if it happens that he dislikes the dentist in both places, he can usually arrange with the district dentist to see someone else.

Dispensary Dental Health Service. The subsystem called dental dispensary care covers most of the population up to the age of nineteen, along with selected groups of adults, amounting to about 6.0 percent of the population, including pregnant and nursing women, military recruits, patients with certain systemic diseases (such as tuberculosis), and persons exposed to professional risks to their dental health. The aim is to screen these priority groups at least once a year, to identify those in need of treatment, and to treat them completely. Dispensary service goes as far as present dental manpower allows. It provides useful data on the work methods and resources that will be necessary for the comprehensive dental service that we envision for the future.

This service is relatively easy to organize for school children, who are captive in the schools. Regular and comprehensive treatment is introduced when the children come to the schools to be inscribed for the first time, which is between the ages of five and six. There, the dentist is present, makes the first screening, and invites those who need treatment to return later on. About 95 percent of school children are reached in this way.

It is, however, considerably more difficult to organize screening programs for preschool children and for adolescents who have moved into jobs or vocational schools. Treatment rates reflect these difficulties. Among preschool children, the rate was only 50 percent in 1975, mainly representing children in kindergarten, while the rate for adolescents varied from 30 to 60 percent, depending on the region of the country.

Primary Prevention

Water fluoridation was introduced about twenty years ago. It is spreading steadily and now reaches about 20 percent of the population. In regions without fluoridated tap water, fluoride tablets are being used, starting with preschool children in kindergartens and creches. About 10 percent of the children are also rinsing with diluted fluoride solutions under the supervision of dental health or teaching personnel.

Consumer Participation

This is an important check on the acceptability of service to the population. Meetings with citizens are arranged at all administrative levels and attended by political and administrative leaders, including ministers of health. The leaders are frequently exposed to critical comments that can become the basis for adjusting the system.

Quality Evaluation

Data are routinely collected by dentists according to a standard system. We follow a number of curative indexes, such as extractions per one hundred simple fillings, number of pulp or root treatments per simple fillings, and the like. We believe that the technical quality achieved by individual dentists has to be checked, along with the performance of the system as a whole. Thus, data are checked and tabulated to permit comparison of the achievements of individual dentists in the same dental health center, of individual dental health centers in the same district, of all districts in a region, and of all regions in the republic. They are published every year, so that practitioners working in the field can see where the performance of their team stands.

SOME RESULTS

In order to know the general state of dental health in Czechoslovakia and to have a baseline for future comparisons, the Ministry of Health organized statewide surveys in 1956 and 1962. The first was a fully randomized survey of a representative sample of the population in the age range two to sixty years; the second covered only the younger part of the population up to the age of twenty. The 1962 survey revealed a medium severity of dental disease among Czechoslovak youth as compared with that of other European countries. Dental caries experience in children ages six to thirteen was 90 percent, and 95 percent in those fourteen to eighteen years. The average number of caries-free teeth (deciduous) in five year olds was fourteen; in twelve year olds (permanent teeth) it was 20.3. The average DMF rate at both five and twelve years was 5.5; by sixteen years of age, it was 9.2; and by nineteen, it was 11.7.

Even in the relatively short time since the 1956 survey, we could see a certain improvement of the dental health state, although the 1962 results in children really reflect the change from a population that had not been treated comprehensively to one that was being treated regularly. The number of fillings in deciduous teeth had doubled at age three and increased by 12 percent at age five. Extractions of three year olds' deciduous teeth dropped by 70 percent and five year olds' by 30 percent. In permanent teeth, the number of fillings increased by 70 percent and 30 percent for ages ten and eighteen respectively. Untreated carious lesions in permanent teeth dropped by 80 percent at age ten and 20 percent at age eighteen.

In 1969, according to data made available to the European Regional Office of the WHO,[1] our children had an average of 1.7 filled permanent teeth at age ten and 6.2 at age fifteen. They also had 0.007 permanent teeth extracted per child at age ten and 0.117 at age fifteen. A 1966 survey showed that about half our children had evidence of gingivitis, whereas the destructive form of periodontal disease did not occur before the age of eighteen. Malocclusion occurred in 27 percent of a random sample of children in 1956–1957. The value of Russell's periodontal index (PI) in a widely distributed but not fully randomized sample of 6,000 adults examined in 1964 was 0.6 for the age range twenty to thirty years, 1.2 for ages thirty to forty, and 1.7 for the group ten years older, with women having worse periodontal health than men.

Using the yardstick of "first things first"—that is, that simple fillings should have highest priority and extractions lowest in dental care delivery—the Czechoslovak dental health service appears to be

Table 13—1.   Some Procedures Performed by the Czechoslovakia Dental Service.

	1972 All Czechoslovakia	1970-1975 Adults	1970-1975 Adolescents
	Percent	Percent	
Simple fillings	46.0	26.8	62.0
Fillings after pulp or root treatment	3.5	4.5	1.9
Extractions	20.0	14.0	2.8
Dentures	4.5	n/a	n/a
Periodontal treatment	9.0	n/a	n/a
Orthodontics	3.0	n/a	n/a
Other	14.0	n/a	n/a

Total: 28 million procedures

Source: Health Statistics in CSSR; dental health service in 1970, 1972, and 1975, *Institute of Health Statistics*, vol. 13: 1971; vol. 15: 1973; and vol. 18: 1976, Prague.

Table 13—2.   Procedures per One Hundred Simple Fillings. *(The dramatic drop in extractions in the military reflects the philosophy of restoring and retaining teeth.)*

	Military 1957	Military 1965	Children 1975
Extractions	7.0	4.1	3.1
Pulp or root treatments	2.6	2.1	1.8

Source: V. Poncova, *Main Trends in our Dental Health Service*. Ministry of Health Current Publications 168 (Prague, 1968). (In Czech)

performing reasonably well, particularly among youth. As Tables 13—1 and 13—2 show, the percentage of simple fillings performed for various age groups in the early 1970s is higher among adolescents than among adults, and the number of extractions and pulpal or root treatments per one hundred fillings appears to be dropping over time.

CONCLUSION

Up till now, I have described features of our dental health service that we think are its strong points. However, our dental service has drawbacks, too.

As in all European countries, there is not enough dental manpower. We need more stomatologists, both to fill vacancies in elementary health areas and to expand the number of specialists in the districts and regions. In addition, the category of stomatological auxiliaries, especially dental hygienists, needs to be extended, and the economy of using medical auxiliaries needs to be examined.

Finally, we need to speed up the use of four-handed dentistry. Four-handed dentistry started only about three years ago in Czechoslovakia and is developing very slowly, due mainly to lack of proper equipment. The government is unable to import expensive, refined equipment. Rather, it must be produced inside the country. Thus, it will be some time before equipment can be substantially upgraded.

Nevertheless, we trust the concept of our health service. We see that its material basis is steadily improving and that its work makes sense. It improves the dental health of our population, and it gives our dental profession the awareness of social function that, I believe, every profession must have in order to enjoy full professional satisfaction.

NOTES

1. *Child Dental Health in Europe.* (WHO, European Regional Office, Copenhagen, 1974).

ABOUT THE AUTHOR

Dr. Jarmil Kostlán is presently the chief research worker in the Institute of Stomatological Research in Prague, Czechoslovakia, where he had previously served as director before accepting an international assignment.

Dr. Kostlán has only recently completed his service as the regional dental officer in the WHO regional office for Europe in Copenhagen. As such he has developed a broad knowledge and acquaintanceship throughout Europe.

In 1966, Dr. Kostlán served as an associate professor of dentistry at the State University of New York, Buffalo.

Dr. Kostlán has received both his M.D. degree and Doctor of Medical Sciences degree from Charles University in Prague.

His present address is: Institute of Stomatological Research, Vinohradska 48, 120 60 Prague 2, Czechoslovakia.

Chapter 14

Notes on Dental Care
Delivery in Other
Eastern European Countries

Dr. Jarmil Kostlán

The concepts of health service in all the Eastern European socialist countries are much alike, though each plays variations on the same theme. In the following notes, I will point to the main differences between the Czechoslovak system and the systems in other Eastern European countries. The figures cited are from 1969 and 1970—unfortunately, the most recent available. Dentist to population ratios are noted in parentheses.

In the *Soviet Union* (1:2,200), the concept of dental health service and the basic set of priorities followed is very similar to those in Czechoslovakia. A special category of dental therapist is used in the USSR. These are trained in vocational schools and on the subuniversity level and used in the dental health service whenever there is a lack of university-trained stomatologists. At the same time, the therapists are encouraged to undertake additional education and to become stomatologists.

The USSR has been very active in water fluoridation since around 1960. At the present time, some twenty million inhabitants are receiving fluoridated water.

The *German Democratic Republic* (1:2,200) has a dental health service of the type typical for socialist countries. Every year, about half the population seeks dental treatment, which is delivered in state run dental offices and polyclinics. About 1,500 private dental practitioners are integrated with the service system. Great emphasis is put on comprehensive and regular treatment of children and adolescents. Water fluoridation was introduced in 1959 and covers one million inhabitants; by 1985, the GDR plans to cover half the population.

In *Poland* (1:2,200), the concept of dental service is similar to that in Czechoslovakia, including the preferential treatment of children. Fluoridated water is available to 5 percent of the population. A particular feature of the Polish dental health service is the dental cooperatives, which offer dental treatment to paying patients; unfortunately, I do not know the details of their functions, administration, and financing.

Hungary (1:3,500–4,000) does not rely on water fluoridation for primary prevention, but it is checking the effectiveness of salt fluoridation in an interesting way, and fluoride tablets are being distributed. Private practice is relatively larger in Hungary than in other Eastern European countries and covers about 25 percent of the total volume of dental service. Every practitioner who fulfills his duty to work six hours a day in government service can engage in private practice.

In *Romania* (1:3,200), water fluoridation has been introduced in one town, but its use has not spread further. Children are treated preferentially, and their dental treatment includes a comprehensive orthodontic regulation. Dental auxiliaries have a relatively high education level. In Romania, as well as in Bulgaria, private practice has been eliminated.

In *Bulgaria* (1:2,500), preferential treatment of children is well organized and covers all preschool children who attend kindergarten. Bulgaria has many mineral waters that are rich in fluoride and are being used in the prevention of dental caries; plans for regular water fluoridation also exist.

Yugoslavia differs substantially from the overall Eastern European pattern. Its system of service follows the pattern of social security. It is, however, financed from the state budget and administered by the so-called House of Health. This system pays dentists per item of service, with part of the salary being adjustable according to the quality of the dentists' work.

ABOUT THE AUTHOR

Dr. Jarmil Kostlán is presently the chief research worker in the Institute of Stomatological Research in Prague, Czechoslovakia, where he had previously served as director before accepting an international assignment.

Dr. Kostlán has only recently completed his service as the regional dental officer in the WHO regional office for Europe in Copenhagen. As such he has developed a broad knowledge and acquaintanceship throughout Europe.

In 1966, Dr. Kostlán served as an associate professor of dentistry at the State University of New York, Buffalo.

Dr. Kostlán has received both his M.D. degree and Doctor of Medical Sciences degree from Charles University in Prague.

His present address is: Institute of Stomatological Research, Vinohradska 48, 120 60 Prague 2, Czechoslovakia.

✳ *Chapter 15*

Dental Care Delivery in Norway

Dr. Per Baerum

Area: 324,000 square kilometers
Population: 4,000,000
Per Capita Gross National Product: $6,616 (1975)
Life Expectancy: 77.8 years (female); 71.5 years (male)

Total expenditure for health care in Norway in 1976 was 9 percent of GNP or $365 per inhabitant. Of that, 60 percent was for hospitals, 15 percent for other medical care, 16 percent for drugs, and 9 percent for dental care.[1]

The delivery of dental care in Norway is principally a local community responsibility. The country has extensive local self-government through approximately 450 municipalities and nineteen counties, each with the right to impose taxes. Approximately 50 percent of all direct taxes are for local government, 25 percent for central government, and 25 percent for social security contributions.

Local district governments operate public health centers, the Public and School Dental Service, and dental care in institutions for the elderly and chronically ill.

The central government provides some financial support to local governments for dental care and, in addition, supervises the appropriateness of relevant laws and national regulations. Central government is also directly responsible for the education of dentists, dental research, and the provision of dental services to centrally owned special schools, university and special hospitals, the military, and the like.

Dentists in private practice are, broadly speaking, responsible for providing dental care to the adult noninstitutionalized population.

MANPOWER RESOURCES

Dentists

There were 4,160 registered dentists, or 1 to 970 inhabitants, in September 1976. Table 15–1 presents the distribution of dentists in 1970 by region and by type of local community. Approximately 150 dentists were specialists, about half of them orthodontists, a quarter oral surgeons, and the rest periodontists. Assuming that 1973 percentages have remained more or less the same, about 54 percent of all dentists were in private practice and 32 percent worked on salary for central or local governments. However, the lines between private and public practice are not strict. Some 15 percent of private practitioners derived part of their income in 1973 from public dental service, teaching, or work in other institutions.[2] And most dentists in district run incremental programs do some fee for service work.

On graduation from secondary school, dentists are trained in a five year course at the dental faculties of either the University of Oslo or the University of Bergen. The total output of these two dental schools is 125 graduates a year. Applicants usually outnumber student acceptances by two or three to one. Two to three year graduate courses in dental specializations are offered by both dental schools,

Table 15–1.   Norwegian Dentists per 1,000 Inhabitants, (a) by Region and (b) by Local Communities' Major Source of Income and Location, 1970.

(a) By Region	Dentists	Dentist to Population Ratio
Ostlandet (Central)	0.96	1:1,042
Sorlandet (South)	0.80	1:1,250
Vestlandet (West)	0.69	1:1,450
Trondelag (Middle)	0.52	1:1,923
Nord-Norge (North)	0.50	1:2,000
(b) By Source of Income of Local Community	Dentists	Dentist to Population Ratio
Fisheries	0.26	1:3,846
Agriculture	0.38	1:2,632
Agriculture plus industry (central location)	0.44	1:2,273
Industry (central location)	0.66	1:1,515
Services plus industry	0.87	1:1,150
Services plus industry (central location)	1.13	1: 855

Source: Government Printing Office, *The Survey on the Level of Living; Final Report* (Oslo, 1976), p. 28.

while Oslo also offers a one year graduate course in community dentistry.

Auxiliary Personnel

There are only about 120 dental hygienists in Norway, with only forty-five new students being trained annually in the two year courses run by the dental schools. Because dental hygienists are in such short supply, a trend is emerging for "dental health assistants" to be trained locally to do preventive work with children in district run programs. Retired or unemployed nurses, housewives, and the like have been employed by a number of local communities, generally on a part-time basis, after a short training course.

Dental laboratory technicians may either learn in a four and a half year apprenticeship or be trained in a three year course in a vocational school. There are about 700 such technicians.

Ninety percent of Norway's private practitioners employ one chairside assistant, and another six percent employ two or more. There are about 5,000 chairside assistants altogether; they can get their training on the job or in a one year course offered by the dental school in Oslo as well as by a number of vocational schools around the country.

MODE OF PRACTICE

Public Incremental Programs
(School and Public Dental Services)

Norwegian children six to seventeen years old are entitled to free incremental care, financed through taxation and given at some 1,400 Public Dental Service clinics situated in or close to the schools of the country. (Climate generally discourages operation of mobile clinics in Norway; consequently, they are practically nonexistent.) Several local communities have included three to five year old children in the incremental program. Some 30 percent of the total treatment time of the Public Dental Service is for the general adult population, particularly in remote areas where private dentists are scarce or nonexistent. Although fixed fees for adult treatment at the clinics are set unilaterally by the central government, local governments may reduce the fees for special groups such as the chronically ill, the handicapped, and the elderly.

The central or local governments are involved in sharing dental costs. National health insurance contributes to the costs of diagnostic and educative services during pregnancy, to restorative services for youngsters sixteen to nineteen who are not covered by the incremental program, to hemophiliacs, and to certain other groups of chronically ill or handicapped persons.

Hospitals are expected to provide necessary dental care for long-term patients, as well as for general patients whose dental conditions interfere with the treatment for which they were hospitalized.

A 1973 survey in Trøndelag offered further insight into the mode of private practice in Norway. Dentists in Trøndelag reported an average of 63 patients a week and spent more than half their time (51 percent) on restorative work. The rest of their time was spent on denture work (11 percent), crown and bridge work (10 percent), endodontic treatment (4 percent), motivation and health education (4 percent), and tooth extraction (4 percent). While 25 percent of the private dentists operated with a waiting time of more than four weeks for new appointments and had to refer new patients to other dentists, 6 percent had no waiting time at all.[3]

The policy of the central government is that, in principle, dentists' work should be paid by the hour. A national standard set of fees for private practice was introduced in 1976, after negotiations between the dental association and the central government.

The Norwegian Dental Association wanted more uniformity in the fees charged by its members. Since organized efforts to regulate prices and market competition cannot be legally undertaken without the approval of the central government, the national fee scale had to be negotiated with it. A second reason the association wanted the national fee scale was its expected importance as a prerequisite for expanded National Health Insurance covering general dental care, which would probably increase the demand for services from the private sector.

The standard fee for one dentist hour was set at NKr. 200, or about $36, for orthodontic and periodontic treatment, partial denture work, and private dental care for children under the age of ten. At the same time, dentists may choose to charge fixed fees per item for fillings, crowns, bridges, full dentures, oral surgery, and x-rays. These fee schedules will be revised in 1977, after the results of a joint professional-government evaluation are known.

. Net income of solo private practitioners averaged 51 percent of gross income in 1973 and was reported to be $17,560, although income varied with the age of the practitioner and the location of the practice. Middle-aged dentists thirty-six to fifty years old and dentists practicing in Oslo had the highest average net incomes—$18,870 and $18,364, respectively. Four percent of all solo practitioners earned $29,668 or more; 3 percent earned less than $8,726. A 1974 survey indicated that physicians earned, on average, 53 percent more than dentists.

A survey of household expenditures in 1973 disclosed that households with total expenditures of $13,960 or more consumed dental care at a rate of $105 per person, while at the other extreme, households with expenditures of $1,745 or less spent $.87 per person.[4] Much of this is covered by the national insurance program, however, which refunds to the individual consumer, regardless of his income, a fixed amount of money per treatment item, including oral surgery and periodontal and orthodontic treatment. Of the total cost of dental care in 1974, private and public, central and local government paid an estimated 26 percent, national insurance 8 percent, and consumers 66 percent. Central and local government share the cost of the National Health Insurance with the members (compulsory membership) and the employers (a special tax).

PREVENTION

Organized programs for topical application of fluoride through rinsing or brushing have been operated since the mid-1960s. In 1976, they were reaching an estimated 70 percent of the population between six and seventeen. Fluoride toothpaste has been widely used since its introduction around 1970; in 1976, it had well over 60 percent of the market. Of the thirteen and fourteen year old students who were surveyed in Trøndelag in 1973, 86 percent had brushed their teeth with fluoride toothpaste the day before the interview. At the same time, a very fortunate reduction in average sugar consumption—from 40.6 kilos per inhabitant in 1972 to 26 kilos in 1975— has been observed.

Until the 1970s, the incremental programs did not sufficiently emphasize prevention of future disease. Children below the age of six were not being treated. Now many local governments, with financial help from the central government, have developed programs for organized distribution of fluoride tablets. In 1976, 60 percent of some 1,300 public health centers providing general maternity and child preventive services distributed the tablets. Nationwide, sales were sufficient to satisfy the optimum intake of 35 percent of all children up to twelve years old.

Effectiveness has begun to show. In Enebakk in 1976, 58 percent of the five year old participants in the fluoride tablet program had experienced no dental decay, compared to 17 percent of nonparticipants.

FUTURE TRENDS

Parliament in January 1975 agreed in principle to a recommendation from the national government that a reorganization of Norwegian dental services should take place. Major points in the government's proposal were:

1. Each county should develop a plan to meet the needs of all age groups in the population, in priority order, through coordination of the services of the private and public schools, and a national plan should also be prepared;
2. More emphasis should be placed on primary prevention, effectiveness, and efficiency of services;
3. Free dental care should be provided to all children up to the age of eighteen; and,
4. The dental services should become an integrated part of the general health services.[5]

The relationship between local governments and the private sector remains to be decided. Some have suggested that national insurance money for dental services, rather than being refunded to individual consumers, should be channeled to the local government, which could then buy planned services from private practitioners or, if necessary, establish a service of its own to implement the community-planned programs.

Present and future investors of public money are not likely to be indifferent to what happens to their investment once children outgrow the incremental programs. Too often, costs and benefits are related only to easily accountable activities. The assumption that the incremental program improves dental health, not only for children under eighteen but afterward, seems to be left unquestioned. And yet, in 1971, it was found that 55 percent of the twenty year old military recruits from Finnmark, the northernmost county, had not visited a dentist during the previous three years. Consequently—unlike their counterparts from Oslo and the rest of the country (Table 15-2)—they had accumulated a considerable need for treatment. To what extent they had also lost the potential for keeping their teeth throughout life is open for future analysis. Fewer and fewer Norwegians obtain regular dental care as they get older (and/or poorer), as Table 15-3 illustrates. They also lose more and more teeth (see Figure 15-1).

Even the value to children of the incremental program has been questioned. The program has taken good care of the treatment re-

Table 15–2. Selected Utilization and Caries Experience Data for Norwegian Military Recruits, Age 20 in 1970.

| Place of Residence | *Percentage Who Saw Their Dentist* | | *Mean Number of Cavities* | *DMF* |
	During Last Twelve Months	*Three Years or More Ago*		
Oslo	56	15	5.4	19
Finnmark	18	55	20.8	18
National Average	47	19	9.2	19

Source: H. Gimnes, Statistical material from the Armed Forces Dental Service Munnpleien 57, no. 273 (1974): 30-39.

Table 15–3. Percentage of Norwegians Receiving Regular Dental Care During the Last Three Years, by Age and Household Income, 1975.

| Age | *Household Income in Nkr. 1,000* | | | | | |
	0–14.9	*15–29.9*	*30–49.9*	*50–79.9*	*80+*	*Norway*
16–29	61	58	63	72	78	69
30–49	40	46	56	65	72	62
50–66	18	20	27	40	61	37
67+	10	13	23	25	23	17

Source: Central Bureau of Statistics, *Survey of Health 1975*, Weekly Statistical Report No. 16 (Oslo 1977).

quirements of the target groups, but it has until recently demonstrated little success in preventing disease.

Figure 15–2 shows that the number of surfaces requiring filling remained between four and six per child, except for a brief period during and immediately after World War II, when sugar was scarce. As recently as 1973, a survey showed the lifetime caries experience of thirteen to fourteen year olds in Trøndelag to be extremely high.[6] The average DMF score was 12.6, practically identical with what had been observed some thirty years earlier.[7]

Recent years have seen a reduction in required treatment time per child per year and an even more dramatic reduction in average number of tooth surfaces requiring filling (Figure 15–3). DMF rates are also falling, as, for example, in Snasa, Trøndelag (Figure 15–4). It seems reasonable to give much of the credit for this improvement in very recent years to an improved personnel situation. While dentists once (1956–1973) were obliged to serve in the public service

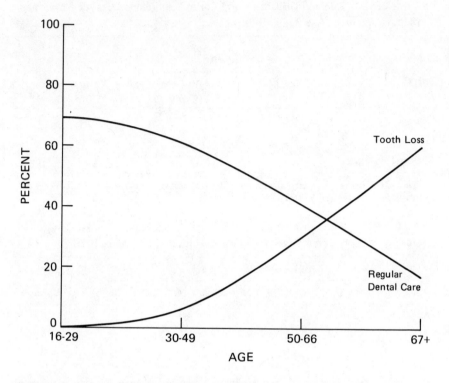

Figure 15–1. Comparison of the Declining Frequency of Regular Dental Care with Increase in Tooth Loss as Related to Age.

Source: Central Bureau of Statistics, *Survey of Health, 1975,* Weekly Statistical Report No. 16 (Oslo 1977).

for a year or two after graduation, competition is now high for positions as district dentists. A permanent, highly motivated, and recently educated young staff must be an invaluable asset to any program.

The former passive acceptance of an ever-increasing need for restorative work, with a focus on activities rather than on end results, now seems largely to have been replaced by an active preventive approach. But the challenge remains to use personnel effectively and efficiently, as well as to involve the parents, schoolteachers, and other health and social service personnel. The essential problem is to see that the children presently in the incremental programs do not end with the same prevalence of tooth loss in their adult years as has been found in the past.

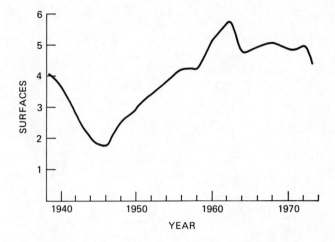

Figure 15–2. Permanent Tooth Surfaces Filled per Year, per Child, Ages Seven to Fifteen, by the Norwegian School Dental Service. *(Except for the war years, when sugar was scarce, caries continued unabated until a recent downturn.)*

Source: The Norwegian Directorate of Health, Dental Division.

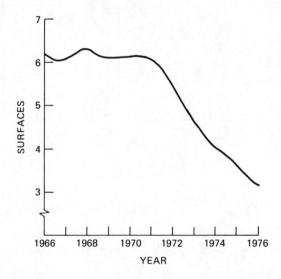

Figure 15–3. Permanent Tooth Surfaces Restored per Child, Ages Six to Seventeen, per Year by the Norwegian Public Dental Service. *(Caries incidence has taken a dramatic downturn since 1970.)*

Source: Central Bureau of Statistics, *Statistical Yearbooks, 1968–1976,* (Oslo).

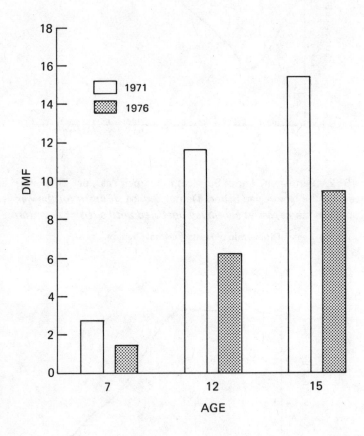

Figure 15-4. Reduction in DMF Teeth at Ages Seven, Twelve, and Fifteen, Snasa, Norway, 1971–1976.

Source: F. Øra, Report on the Public Dental Service in Snasa, Trøndelag (1977; unpublished data).

NOTES

1. Central Bureau of Statistics of Norway, *Survey of Consumer Expenditure 1973* (Oslo: 1975).
2. The Norwegian Dental Association, Survey on Fees in Private Practice, (May 1974; unpublished data).
3. Per Baerum and H. Arnljot, Dentists in Trøndelag—Mode of Practice and Attitudes (in preparation).
4. Central Bureau of Statistics.
5. Ministry of Social Affairs, *Report to Parliament No. 111 (1973-74), On the Public Dental Services* (Oslo, 1974).
6. Per Baerum and H. Arnljot, Oral Health Care in Norway, *Int. Dent. J.* 26 (September 1976: 340-45).
7. G. Toverud, The Influence of War and Postwar Condition in Teeth of Norwegian Schoolchildren, *Milbank Memorial Fund Quarterly* II, 35 (1957): 127.

ABOUT THE AUTHOR

Dr. Per Baerum is the director of the dental division in the Directorate of Health, Ministry of Social Affairs, of Norway. Prior to that he was a consultant to the Ministry Dental Division and an instructor in the Department of Peridontology at the School of Dentistry at the University of Oslo.

Dr. Baerum has also served as the coordinator for Norway in the WHO/USPHS International Collaborative Study reported in Chapter 20. Internationally, he has been a consultant and advisor to WHO as well as to the Federation Dentaire Internationale.

Dr. Baerum received his dental degree (Cand. Odont.) at the University of Oslo in 1953 and his Master's degree in Public Health at the University of Michigan, Ann Arbor, in 1967.

His present address is: Dental Division, Directorate of Health, Ministry of Social Affairs, Oslo-dep., Oslo 1, Norway.

Chapter 16

Dental Care Delivery
in Sweden

Dr. Jan Erik Ahlberg

Area: 480,000 square kilometers
Population: 8,200,000 (1976)
Per Capita Gross National Product: $8,420 (1975)
Life Expectancy: seventy-five years

The picture of the Swedish dental care delivery system is frequently painted either in very somber or very rosy colors. Both color schemes tend to obscure the real situation.

Sweden begins with some very important advantages in mounting a dental care delivery system. First, it is rich; Swedish per capita income is among the highest in the world. Second, there has been a fortunate tendency on the part of the government and the population to give oral care a relatively high priority. And third, the number of dentists is, at 1:1,000, the highest in the world in relation to population and is equaled only by that of Norway. Indeed, I am convinced that the number of dentists in Sweden by the end of this century, when the ratio is likely to be 1:500, will prove to be excessive.

There is, furthermore, great need for an effective delivery system. Very high incidence of caries and periodontal disease is typical of the population, among the newest groups of immigrants as well as among native-born Swedes.

The Swedish population receives its dental care either from private practitioners or through the National Dental Service, each of which encompasses approximately half of the 8,000 dentists in Sweden. The National Dental Service is charged primarily with caring for all children from birth to age nineteen. About one-third of all adults in

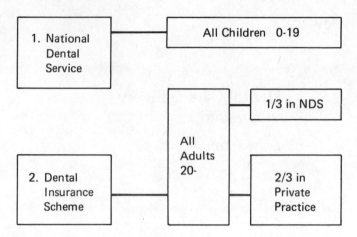

Figure 16–1. Administrative Responsibility of the Swedish National Dental Service to Treat All Children and One-third of the Adults.

Sweden are also cared for under the NDS. The remaining adults are treated in private practices, but part of their fees are paid under the Swedish Dental Insurance scheme (Figure 16–1).

There are about 1.3 chairside assistants per dentist, an adequate number and one that is expected to increase to 1.5 per dentist in the future. The number of dental hygienists is very limited, however, and New Zealand type dental nurses or expanded duty auxiliaries do not exist.

THE NATIONAL DENTAL SERVICE

The National Dental Service is not administered by the state but by the so-called "Landsting," or county councils, whose main responsibilities are medical and dental care, for which they have autonomous power to raise taxes. Since the late 1930s, all the county councils have gradually built up dental services, primarily for children. In some of the biggest cities, clinics exist in schools, but the great majority are neighborhood clinics voluntarily erected by the county councils and subsidized by the state for equipment and running costs on condition that school children receive regular treatment, systematically class by class, free of charge. Treatment of adults is allowed in these clinics according to a fixed scale of fees, established by the state, that is supposed to cover the real costs of treatment.

Today, Sweden has a network of dental clinics spread all over the country. The standard of buildings and equipment is generally high. Successive modernization of buildings and equipment is taking place all over the country. The county councils may even have been more generous in the planning of accessory space, for instance, than most private practitioners would have been. There seems to be little difference in the average standard of equipment between private practice and the National Dental Service. Equipment used in both systems is rather similar to what one finds in the United States, except, perhaps, that handpieces and syringes are placed so they can be reached from above instead of from the side when the dentist is seated.

The dentist in the National Dental Service works mainly on a salary system. In addition, however, most receive a bonus that is based on a sort of fee for service calculation for the treatment of both children and adults. In 1975, the average income of employed dentists in the middle of the promotion scale was about $19,500. The usual beginning income was about $13,500.

When introduced, it was anticipated that the National Dental Service would be able to meet its treatment targets after a relatively short period of time and with a moderate number of dentists. This turned out to be a gross misjudgment. Apart from such unpredictable factors as an initial delay due to World War II and soaring birth rates during the 1940s, a lack of proper preliminary epidemiologic investigations led to a serious underestimate of the need for dental care among Swedish children. On average, each child requires almost two hours in the dental chair per year. It was to take more than thirty years, and a massive input of dentists, before the original targets were met as far as children were concerned.

But the original targets have been met. It is a considerable achievement to be able to treat regularly more than 90 percent of the children between six and sixteen years of age. In fact, practically all children in this age group receive complete treatment over any fifteen month period. Nearly 50 percent of children between three and five years of age and one-third of the adolescents between seventeen and nineteen received complete treatment in 1975, and these figures have increased since then.

But by now the National Dental Service has revised its goals. A major dental reform took place in Sweden on July 1, 1973. As noted previously, the National Dental Service is now charged with the complete treatment of all children and adolescents between birth and nineteen years of age. They will also provide approximately one-third of adult treatment. The service will still be run by the county councils, but this is now a statutory, rather than a voluntary, task. Services for children have been given high priority, and it is expected that the county councils will be able to meet their targets by the early 1980s.

Adult treatment under the National Dental Service has had only mixed success. A number of adults, particularly of low income and in the rural communities, have had access to dental treatment that might not otherwise have been available to them; this is particularly true for full denture wearers. But the intention to create, in the National Dental Service, a cheaper source of adult dental care open to all has failed. The service was never designed to take care of a large proportion of the adult population. The idea that it should still, in principle, be open to all adults might have worked reasonably well if the scale of fees had been allowed to follow the actual cost of dental treatment. During the 1950s and 1960s, however, the Swedish government allowed the fee schedule to lag further and further behind real costs, with the result that heavy demand—particularly for more complicated, costly, and time-consuming treatment—forced a limitation on the number of patients who could be treated.

Furthermore, the service has not proved to be cost-effective. Studies have indicated that the time taken to complete various items of treatment is, on average, the same for private practitioners and dentists in the National Dental Service. A slight difference to the disadvantage of the dental service, which needed to spend more time on administrative matters, has probably been eliminated by the introduction of more government-required paper work in private practice.

PRIVATE PRACTICE

Private practice caters at present to 80—85 percent of the dental care of adults and is expected to cover at least two-thirds of the adult population in the future. Most private practitioners work in solo practice or in a practice of two dentists. Real group practice is rare, although some 1,650 private dentists, more than one in five, and 400 physicians have joined the Group Practice Corporation. This corporation is not a group practice in the traditional sense, but it offers many of the advantages of one and contributes significantly to the high quality of private dental services in Sweden. The corporation also provides efficiencies of scale in capital management and considerable administrative rationalization. It employs more than 8,000 persons, including auxiliary personnel and the like. The potential for innovation in such a corporation is great. In 1976, more than 80 percent of the dentists in the corporation devoted one week or more to continuing education, for example. Many of them subscribe to a five year plan in which continuing education in the various main areas of dental science is arranged in sequence.

For most of the postwar period, the supply of dentists was adequate for the treatment provided. In fact, by the mid-1960s, it had become obvious that there was a considerable—and rapidly increasing—spare capacity for dental treatment. Costly reforms in the medical field threatened to deprive dentistry of financial resources and hampered the expansion of children's dentistry in the National Dental Service. Furthermore, potential demand from adults was not materializing, due primarily to financial reasons.

This situation provided the impetus for the second aspect of the 1973 dental reform, which was to establish a comprehensive dental insurance plan to meet the needs of all the population. This insurance, which came into full effect from January 1974, is part of the well-known Swedish social insurance scheme, which also covers allowances for medical expenses, sickness benefits, parental insurance, and pensions.

NATIONAL DENTAL INSURANCE

The dental insurance includes all forms of treatment, including preventive measures, given by dentists in both private practice and the National Dental Service. The vast majority of private practitioners have contracted with the insurance scheme. They are not compelled to do so, but only a very limited number have preferred to contract out.

Under this scheme, the patient pays half the cost of his dental treatment up to a limit of 500 Swedish crowns in the course of any one treatment period. When treatment is more expensive, the patient pays only 25 percent of the cost above 1,000 crowns. The insurance always assumes 75 percent of the cost for prophylaxis and for full dentures.

If a dentist decides to work for the insurance system, he is not entitled to treat patients on a purely private basis, charging higher fees. He must adhere to a rather complicated scale of fees. Standard items of treatment are given one fixed fee. Where the time needed for treatment might vary considerably, items of treatment have three, or even four, different fee levels, depending on the difficulty of the individual case. Where the time needed for treatment is particularly varied, a fixed fee per hour is applicable. Any necessary technical appliances are figured separately from the dentist's fee for treatment.

To the private practitioner, the insurance works as a fee for service system. The patient pays his part of the cost directly to the dentist, who then sends monthly invoices to the local insurance office for the rest of the cost. The net income of the average private practitioner, calculated on the same number of working hours as for the average employed dentist, was approximately $22,000 in 1975, in comparison to an average industrial wage of about $10,000.

The total cost for dental care in 1974 amounted to about $346 million. Out of this, the adult patients themselves paid about $110 million, the insurance scheme $166 million. The cost for the treatment of children amounted to roughly $70 million. The average cost per adult patient was about $80, per child about $55. Of course, the money for the dental insurance scheme does not come out of the air. Employers and self-employed persons pay most of it—about 85 percent—while direct taxation covers the remaining 15 percent.

It is too early to make an evaluation of the dental insurance system. Complete statistics exist only for its first year. On the face of it, the insurance system has tended initially to create almost as many problems as it solves. This is because demand has exploded. In contrast to the situation in the midsixties, a shortage of dental resources has developed. One consequence is a long wait for appointments among adults not previously regular patients of any dentist. The time for delivery of technical appliances has increased far beyond the reasonable, causing disorganization in the dental offices to the point of being harmful to the patient. Furthermore, with the enormous increase in demand from adults, the expansion—or even the maintenance—of the capacity for children's dentistry was endangered, and it became necessary to restrict the increase of private practitioners in order to safeguard the children's program.

It is impossible to know how long these problems will remain, although the worst shortages may soon be over. A great number of adults have now had their needs for crown and bridge prostheses and full dentures satisfied.

PREVENTIVE MEASURES

Two specific features of the Swedish system have contributed greatly to improved dental health.

Fluoride Mouth Rinses

Water with a natural fluoride content is rare in Sweden. Artificial fluoridation of water is, for the time being, prohibited by law as a result of a surprise action by the Swedish Parliament some years ago. Although this may change under the new government, other methods of fluoridation are already in use and widely accepted by the public.

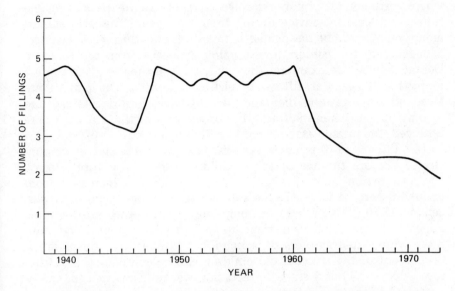

Figure 16—2. Number of Fillings Placed per Child by the School Dental Service in Goteborg, Sweden, 1938–1973. *(The dramatic drop since 1960 is credited to the fluoride mouthrinse program. The decrease during World War II reflects a drop in sugar consumption.)*

One method, started almost twenty-five years ago and now well established, is collective mouthrinsing with 0.2 fluoride solution. This is organized through the schools. All children, in all types of schools, now rinse their mouths every two weeks with the solution. In the beginning, the teachers were responsible for supervising the rinsing; nowadays, specially trained assistants organize the mouthrinsings.

A number of investigations have demonstrated the beneficial effects of these mouthrinses. In Goteborg, Sweden's second largest city, for example, the number of fillings per child per year has decreased from five in 1940 to two in 1973 (Figure 16—2). Again, in Norrbotten, the most northerly county in Sweden, the number of DMF teeth among sixteen year olds decreased from 19.8 in 1962 to 10.5 in 1971; among eighteen year old men, the decrease was from 40 in 1958 to 29 in 1973.

Maternity Center Activities
Perhaps even more important than the mouthrinses is the very early involvement of children in the so-called maternity centers

where virtually all children receive medical examinations, vaccinations, and medical advice during their first year. This also started many years ago, but has gained momentum only during the last decade. Most of the centers now employ a dentist from the National Dental Service. He examines the child, once at the age of six to nine months and again at fifteen to eighteen months. The parents are given advice regarding diet and oral hygiene. Fluoride tablets are recommended. When malformation or diseases of the oral cavity are observed, the infants are referred to a dental clinic.

The effects of this advisory activity have been clearly demonstrated. Before the age of three, children rarely show tooth decay. The proportion of caries-free three year olds has increased from about 20 percent in the 1940s and 1950s to a range of 50 to 75 percent in 1970 (Table 16—1). Among five year olds, the corresponding increase is from 5 to 10 percent up to 25 to 40 percent. In communities where the treatment of preschool children is well consolidated, 30 percent of the six year old children can be completely free from tooth decay. (When I started practicing twenty-five years ago, barely 1 percent of six year olds were caries-free.)

In addition, the localization of decay has changed. Decay of the buccal and lingual surfaces, as well as of the incisors, is seen less often. Only decay of the aproximal surfaces occurs among five and six year olds. This means, of course, that the number of children with treatment difficulties is considerably lower.

Table 16—1. Caries-free Three Year Old Children in Sweden, Reported by Survey and Year.

Survey	Year	Percentage
Roos	1944	17
Sundvall-Hagland	1955	17
Sjoberg and Hedlin	1964	23
Gothardsson, et al.	1970	61
Rosenkranz	1970	41
Holm and Arvidsson	1970	55
Rosenkranz	1972	67
Bjorne	1973	75
Goteburg Faculty	1974	74

Plaque Control

An exciting experimental program for plaque control in children is reported on in Chapter 21. It is not yet a full-fledged government program, but initial results from the pilot project are most promising.

CONCLUSIONS

To sum up, I am confident that, within a decade, the dental care delivery system will cater for the need of all children and adolescents and, in the slightly longer term, will meet almost the total demand from adults. But this is not necessarily due to the delivery system proper. The relative success of recent children's dentistry, for example, is to a great extent due to the systematic application of preventive measures. It is not certain—in fact, it is rather unlikely—that an organizational design like the one in Sweden is necessary to achieve the same results.

Sweden shares with most industrialized countries the problem that dental care has been too much reparative and too little preventive. I would be happy if I could convey to you the strength of my conviction, based on Swedish experience, that the first obligation of the politicians, as well as the leaders of the profession, is to implement successful oral prevention. Only after that is done, can one consider how to make prevention tally with the existing delivery system and other local conditions. Indeed, it will be interesting to follow to what extent the inclusion and, in fact, the special support of preventive measures in the insurance scheme will affect the structure of dental care on a long-term basis, particularly if we succeed in using dental assistants and the like to perform most preventive tooth cleaning.

ABOUT THE AUTHOR

Dr. Ahlberg is presently the executive director of the Federation Dentaire Internationale, with headquarters in London. Prior to his rather recent acceptance of this international assignment, he was executive director of the Swedish Dental Federation. As such he had a good deal to do with helping direct Sweden's efforts in the delivery of dental care as well as with formulating policy for the future.

Dr. Ahlberg received his dental degree (Leg. Tandlakare) from the Faculty of Odontology at the Karolinska Institute in Stockholm.

His present address is: 64 Wimpole Street, London W1m 8AL, England.

❋ *Chapter 17*

Notes on Dental Care Delivery in The Netherlands

Dr. Jan Erik Ahlberg

Area: 36,757 square kilometers
Population: 13,800,000 (1976)
Per Capita Gross National Product: $5,250 (1974)
Life Expectancy: seventy-four years

In the Netherlands, the dentist to population ratio is approximately 1:3,500. The number of dental hygienists is limited.

The school dental service works according to different alternatives. Either the school dentist performs only the examination and refers the child to a private dentist or he or she carries out the treatment as well as the examination.

The national dental insurance scheme covers about 70 percent of the population. Its most interesting and unusual feature is the dental fitness card—a sort of entrance fee to the dental delivery system. It works as follows:

Patients who are not dentally "fit" get necessary x-rays, extractions, and other surgical treatment free of charge but must pay part of the cost of their restorative dental work. On completion of the treatment, the patient is issued a "dental fitness card," which is dated, and is told to return within six months. Once the patient achieves the status of being dentally fit, x-rays, examinations, simple fillings, root canal treatment, and prophylactic treatment are free to the patient, though he is still obliged to pay part of the cost for a fixed or a full or partial denture. If the patient fails to return within six months, however, he is again regarded as being not dentally fit, and he has to get dental treatment at his own expense before he is issued a new dental fitness card.

ABOUT THE AUTHOR

Dr. Ahlberg is presently the executive director of the Federation Dentaire Internationale, with headquarters in London. Prior to his rather recent acceptance of this international assignment, he was executive director of the Swedish Dental Federation. As such he had a good deal to do with helping direct Sweden's efforts in the delivery of dental care as well as with formulating policy for the future.

Dr. Ahlberg received his dental degree (Leg. Tandlakare) from the Faculty of Odontology at the Karolinska Institute in Stockholm.

His present address is: 64 Wimpole Street, London W1m 8AL, England.

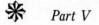 *Part V*

Two "Continental" Systems

The juxtaposition of two dental care delivery systems, China and the United States, points up the gulf of difference in the political systems between the two countries.

As Dr. Harold Hillenbrand noted in his summary statement (Chapter 4), there is very little that U.S. dentists or the government of the United States can learn from the dental delivery system in China. On the other hand, China has learned a good deal about the practice of dentistry and about dental education from North Americans. Someday, in reciprocity, Western dentistry may find some value in the physiotherapy, acupuncture, or use of drugs today favored by Chinese stomatologists.

Through the use of auxiliary personnel, China is attempting to reach a segment of its overwhelming population that had never before seen a dentist other than a village tooth puller. In striving to achieve this goal, they may well outdistance the United States, where dental care is also not received by a significant portion of the population.

✳ *Chapter 18*

Dental Care Delivery in the People's Republic of China

Dr. John I. Ingle

> Area: 9,583,000 square kilometers
> Population: 900,000,000 (estimated)
> Per Capita Gross National Product: $320 (estimated)
> Life Expectancy: sixty-two years

Delivery of health care, and particularly dental care, in China is closely tied to the distribution of its massive population (95 percent of the people live in the eastern half of the nation), as well as to accidents of weather and geography peculiar to that country. Eighty percent of China's population is rural, but most of it is grouped into 70,000 communes, with populations ranging from 10,000 to 80,000. The remaining 20 percent of the population is crowded into enormous cities, with Shanghai (population: twelve million) being the largest; fifteen other cities have more than one million inhabitants. This demography makes collectivization of dental care possible and natural, as well as politically advisable (Figures 18–1 and 18–2).

"In medical and health work, put the stress on the rural areas," read Mao Tse Tung's dictum of June 26, 1965. Chairman Mao went on to emphasize prevention, a priority established at the first Chinese National Health Congress in 1950. This early congress also set the pattern for the future, with an insistence that "health workers must serve the workers, peasants and soldiers," and that "traditional Chinese doctors (*zhong yi*) be integrated with the 'Western' doctors (*ziyi*) as part of the mass movement."

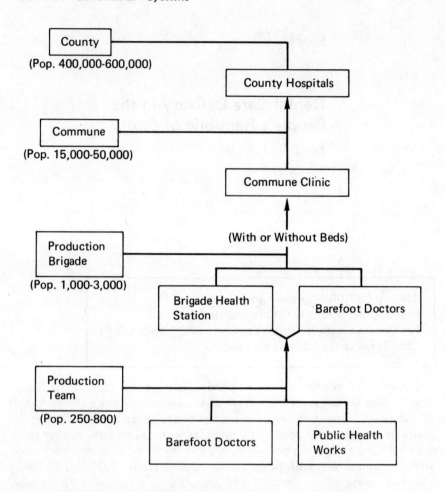

Figure 18—1. Rural Health Care and its Referral System in China.

Source: T.W. Hu, *An Economic Analysis of Cooperative Medical Services in the People's Republic of China*, John E. Fogarty International Center, DHEW Publ. No. (NIH) 75—672, (Washington, D.C.: U.S. Government Printing Office, 1975).

But a health care delivery system with these priorities requires unheard of numbers of health care providers to practice in the countryside. With only a few Western type physicians and dentists in China, the revolutionary Chinese government rapidly developed innovative forms of health care. The village empiricists—acupuncturists, herbalists, and bone setters—were integrated into the Western medical mode, and the village tooth pullers were incorporated into a broadened system for dental care.

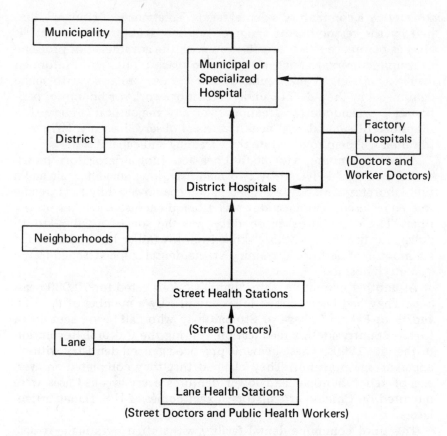

Figure 18-2. Urban Health Care and Its Referral System in China.

Source: T.W. Hu, *An Economic Analysis of Cooperative Medical Services in the People's Republic of China*, John E. Fogarty International Center, DHEW Publ. No. (NIH) 75-672, (Washington, D.C.: U.S. Government Printing Office, 1975).

DENTAL HEALTH WORKERS
AND BAREFOOT DOCTORS

In addition to Westernizing the traditionalists, one of the most creative Chinese innovations was to develop a new class of paramedical worker, the "barefoot doctor," trained to deliver care at the production brigade level. It is estimated that over 800,000 of these paramedics are presently functioning in China.

The dental counterpart of the barefoot doctor is the "dental health worker," often a converted rural dental empiricist who formerly worked in the streets, now further trained and brought indoors to care for a community's dental needs. Treatment, of course, is limited by the restriction of training, but the dental health worker is able, as before, to extract teeth (now with the advantages of procaine or acupuncture analgesia), as well as to place fillings and preformed stainless crowns. Some dental health workers are trained to make dentures, but they do not undertake bridgework; orthodontic, periodontic, or endodontic treatment; or any major oral surgery. Descriptions of some dental health workers observed on my 1973 visit to China will help to illustrate their training and capabilities:

At one commune, with 26,000 peasants (not a derogatory term), dental care was delivered by two men using one ancient chair and a tiny laboratory. An old-fashioned handpiece powered by foot treadle was being used. The cuspidor was a blood-encrusted bucket on the floor. The dental worker on duty was the son of a village tooth puller; he had learned this "skill" from his father but had also had six months of additional training at the dental clinic attached to the "county" hospital.

At another commune, three dental workers cared for 70,000 peasants. They had been trained in six months by a member of the University of Peking College of Stomatology who had been "sent down to the countryside for reeducation" during the Cultural Revolution of the late 1960s. These peasants practiced general dentistry with no apparent age priorities. They claimed that they completed an average of ten full upper and lower dentures every week. Cases were mounted on Chinese articulators—exact copies of U.S. Hanau articulators.

The third commune dental facility was staffed by a male–female team. We westerners "naturally" assumed the man was in charge, but in this case, the woman was the dental worker and the male was her assistant, called a dental nurse by the Chinese.

The barefoot doctors also deliver some dental care in remote regions where no dental workers are available. Each is equipped with a tooth extraction kit. After three months to a year of health care training, the barefoot doctor is sent into the field with a manual that, among other things, illustrates how to make oral injections and extract root tips. The manual also illustrates how to perform tubal ligations, deliver babies, perform appendectomies, and repair facial clefts. All of these "lower case" health workers—the barefoot doctors and dental health workers—are involved in continuing education, returning to the county or provincial level for refresher and further training programs.

DENTAL TECHNICIANS

The next level of dental care personnel, above the dental health worker, is the dental technician, not to be confused with the dental laboratory technician known in other countries as well as in China. Dental technicians are trained for six months to a year in dental "schools." At the end of their training, they are qualified, by Chinese standards, to deliver general dental care—simple restorative and periodontal work, root canal therapy, full denture prosthetics, and simple extractions. It would appear that most serve an "internship" in clinics, under the supervision of a stomatologist, before serving on their own. They are backed up by dental nurses and laboratory technicians, however, and are expected to return periodically for refresher courses.

The Chinese have not released figures on the number of dental technicians presently practicing in China, nor have they revealed how many dental schools are operating in the country. There are said to be ten schools in Shanghai alone, so one would have to assume that this is a widespread educational movement graduating thousands of "technicians" each year. It soon becomes apparent that these technicians are delivering the bulk of China's general dental care.

THE STOMATOLOGISTS

Western type dentistry in China is comparatively new, the first dental "college" (as distinct from the dental schools for technicians) having been established in 1916 at West China Union University, Chengtu, Szechwan Province. Canadian-born Dr. Ashley Lindsay started this college, and Dr. Gordon Agnew, emeritus professor of the University of California, San Francisco, was a pioneering member of the faculty.

From this meager start only sixty years ago, education in stomatology has grown very slowly in China. Today, there are only five faculties graduating dentists to serve some 900 million people. Quite obviously, dentists are limited in number and in the services they perform.

Chinese stomatologists (as they prefer to be called) serve primarily as the administrators of dental care delivery programs, overseeing the practicing dental technicians. In addition, stomatologists serve as the diagnosticians of complex cases and as oral, maxillofacial, and plastic surgeons; they plan and oversee orthodontic treatment; carry out complex restorative, fixed prosthodontic, periodontic, and endodontic procedures; and, of course, serve as faculty.

Stomatologists also have major responsibility for most dental care delivered in large clinics, called dental prevention and treatment centers. Again, it is not known how many of these centers there are. Each dental prevention and treatment center has four divisions: children's dentistry, adult dentistry, oral surgery, and prevention, with prevention appearing to be an extramural as well as intramural responsibility involving schools and home care. Dentists head each section.

One center visited in Manchuria had a professional staff of seventy-five people (sixty-five of them were females) made up of ten stomatologists and sixty-five dental technicians. The director was a female stomatologist, though the inevitable vice chairman of the Revolutionary Committee, not a dentist, was a male. (This "most responsible person" in each organization ties the operation to the government and the party but does not appear to oversee professional performance or standards. Surprisingly, these party functionaries are paid much less than the dental hierarchy.)

There do not appear to be dental clinics in the primary or secondary schools or dental facilities in the small neighborhood health clinics. Every hospital in China seems to have an outpatient dental service, however, and some of the secondary and tertiary health centers have inpatient dental services as well. Stomatologists professionally staff all inpatient and most outpatient hospital dental services and are heavily assisted by dental nurses as well as clerks, sterilizing personnel, porters, and cleaning persons. One must remember that China's economy is labor-intensive and that lavish use of workers is the norm. No dental hygienists, per se, are apparent although dental technicians and even dental nurses (assistants) serve in this capacity.

The hospital associated with a huge iron and steel collective in An Shan, Manchuria, is typical. There is a professional staff of seven—five stomatologists and two technicians—to man the outpatient and inpatient services. They see over one hundred patients a day. The director of the dental service, which was attached to the eye, ear, nose, and throat service, was a very sophisticated, self-trained oral surgeon who spoke English very competently even though he had never been outside China.

Oral surgeons in China appear to be restricted only by their skills, not by some artificial barrier imposed by other disciplines in medicine. The most notable example I encountered was full body plastic surgery being performed by a self-trained oral surgeon for a patient who was burned over 70 percent of her body. The oral surgeon had been called upon to relieve the cicatrices attaching the lower lip to the chin and the chin to the chest wall. Over the period of a year, the oral surgeon had also relieved the scarring in the antecubital fossa to straighten out the arms and was straightening out the fingers that had been drawn up into claws. The Chinese place great importance on the dignity of the individual, including their appearance. Much emphasis is also placed on correcting facial clefts and disfigurement or crippling malocclusions.

Orthodontists, some trained years ago in the United States, rank equally with oral surgeons in the Chinese dental hierarchy. The Chinese are attempting to treat orthodontically great numbers of children, usually employing removable appliances, so that adjustments can be made more easily in the event the youngster moves to a different location. One has the feeling, however, that very few peasant children have their teeth straightened.

COMPENSATION

Compensation for dental personnel appears to be fairly well standardized nationwide along the lines shown in Table 18—1. Lower level personnel are paid about the same as the peasants and barefoot doctors—35 to 40 yuan monthly.

All second level dental workers have the privilege of escalating from their positions to higher levels. If recommended by their fellow workers, and with more education, dental nurses and "workers" may move up to technicians, technicians to stomatologists, and general stomatologists into the dental specialties. Health science specialists are among the elite in a society claiming to be proletarian. They receive higher salaries and perquisites not available to lesser beings— chauffeured transportation, better housing, the right to hire servants, and so forth. The dental specialist salaries appear to range from 200 yuan a month up to 340 yuan for the dean of a dental school. Medical salaries are comparable. (For comparison, Chairman Mao was said to have received 450 yuan a month.)

A director of a dental prevention and treatment center receives twice what a third year stomatologist receives, whereas the party functionary in a clinic, the vice chairman of the Revolutionary Committee, earns about one-third less than the dental director.

Many professional families have a combined income of as much as 400 yuan a month. Out of this, they pay 7 yuan for a three bedroom apartment with utilities, about 15 yuan monthly for food for each, and 40 yuan a month for an "aunty," a housemaid who appears to be one of the few remaining examples of free enterprise in China. A family of four with a maid would, therefore, spend about 110 yuan a month out of 400 yuan income. The remaining 290 yuan could be

Table 18-1.   Comparative Salaries for Dental Personnel, People's Republic of China, 1973. *(Commune dental workers are paid the same as field hands, as are barefoot doctors.)*

1.00 yuan comparable to $0.50 U.S.

Faculty of Stomatology	per month
Dean	340.00Y
Professor of Oral Surgery (foreign trained)	269.00Y
Assistant Professor, Pedodontics	215.00Y
Chairman of the Revolutionary Committee	100.00Y

Department of Stomatology (Hospital)	
Associate Professor of Oral Surgery	200.00Y
Director of Clinics	70.00Y
Instructor	
First year	51.5 Y
Second year	61.5 Y
Third year	68.5 Y

Dental Prevention and Treatment Center	
Director	140.00Y
Dentist	
First year	56.00Y
Second year	66.00Y
Third year	78.00Y
Dental Technician	45.00Y to 70.00Y
Dental Nurse	35.00Y to 45.00Y
Laboratory Technician	45.00Y to 60.00Y
Dental "worker" commune	30.00Y to 40.00Y

Comparison	
Factory worker, soldier, or "cadre"	70.00Y
Commune "peasant"	30.00Y to 40.00Y

used to buy clothes, bicycles, television, radio, even a piano, and eventually a camera. No one but the state may own an automobile, however. Part of savings is banked (at 2.5 percent interest) for vacations and out of habit. Anyone who owned their home before the revolution continues to live in it rent free. There is, of course, no malpractice liability.

With health care, education, and retirement assured, Chinese professionals have no need for a savings or retirement program. They work for, and are compensated by, the state throughout their education and careers; they are supported in retirement by the state, and they are buried by the state. No taxes are paid by the people, and salaries come from the "profit" each unit of the state makes in its operation.

PAYMENT FOR HEALTH SERVICES

For a communist nation, China uses peculiar systems of payment for health services rendered—"labor medical insurance" (LMI) for factory workers and "cooperative medical services" (CMS) for the rural peasants. CMS is voluntary. I had no difficulty obtaining copies of a fairly standard fee schedule used nationwide by government clinics and hospitals (Table 18—2).

When the patient's dental work (or hospital stay) is completed, the patient pays the fee and is given a chit that he turns in to CMS at his commune or LMI at his collective. He is then compensated by the organization according to their program—some at the rate of 100 fen on the yuan, others at 80 percent. Dental fees for the peasants appear to be at half fee, one of the perquisites (such as free housing and food for half cost) to improve the lot of the rural workers.

Each month, each worker or peasant pays 10 to 20 fen (comparable to 5 to 10 cents) into the collective health care fund, which is then used to compensate those who utilize the system. Dependents have to pay half of their health care charges, so they often wait until they become ill before joining the collective fund. Government workers (called "cadres"), soldiers, students, and retired persons are treated free in government clinics.

The Chinese are willing to work on foreigners using the same fee schedule. I observed a visiting Indonesian (Chinese) school teacher, for example, who received a full upper denture over a cast lower partial for only 22 yuan (U.S. $11.00), a tenth of what it would have cost in Jakarta. The quality was excellent. A U.S. television cameraman had his teeth cleaned for three yuan (U.S. $1.50) and was told they would make him a three unit bridge, with root canal therapy for one abutment, for less than 20 yuan (U.S. $10.00). The abutments would be preformed stainless steel crowns with plastic facings.

Table 18–2. Dental Fee Structure, People's Republic of China, 1973. *(Commune peasants pay half these fees; for example, 10 yuan ($5.00 U.S.) for full upper and lower dentures.)*

1.00 yuan comparable to $0.50 U.S.

Restorative

Amalgams
Deciduous	0.30Y to 0.50Y
Permanent	0.50Y to 1.00Y
Resins	0.50Y to 1.00Y
Inlay (white metal)	2.00Y
Temporary cement	0.30Y

Endodontics

Mummification
Deciduous	1.00Y
Permanent	2.00Y
Root canal filling	
Anterior	2.00Y
Posterior	3.00Y

Periodontics

Scaling and medication per visit	0.20Y to 0.30Y
Gingivectomy	1.00Y
Flap operation	1.00Y
Densensitization and selective grinding, per tooth	0.10Y
Temporary splint	
Floss	0.50Y
Wire	1.00Y

Prosthetics

Fixed
Chrome-cobalt crown	2.00Y
Open-faced crown	2.50Y
Acrylic jacket crown	2.50Y
Post and coping crown	4.00Y
Three-unit bridge	8.00Y
Four-unit bridge	9.70Y
Occlusal splint	5.00Y

Removable

One-tooth replacement	2.00Y
Three-tooth replacement	4.10Y
Cast chrome-cobalt, lower	15.40Y
Upper tissue bar—three clasps	7.00Y
Cast, free end saddles	15.60Y
Skeleton cast, five clasps	20.00Y
Full upper denture	10.00Y
Full lower denture	10.00Y

Orthodontics

Full treatment	4.00Y

Oral Surgery

Extractions
Molar tooth	1.00Y
Premolar tooth	0.80Y
Anterior tooth	0.60Y
Deciduous tooth	0.40Y
Impaction	1.50Y to 2.00Y
Tumor surgery	15.00Y
Fracture reduction	15.00Y
Cleft palate repair	10.00Y
Hare lip repair	4.00Y

Comparisons

Appendectomy	12.00Y
Tubal ligation	7.00Y
Daily hospital charge	1.00Y
Vasectomy	3.00Y
Heart-lung machine surgery	100.00Y

DENTAL EDUCATION

In 1972, education for a stomatologist (and a physician) was limited to three years. Initial requirements for entry are graduation from "high school" followed by service of two years "in the countryside" or as a member of the armed forces, a factory worker, or barefoot doctor.

Prior to the Cultural Revolution, which began in 1968, the courses in stomatology or medicine were six years. Universities were closed during the Cultural Revolution and reopened with new curricula that reduced required course time by 50 percent. Some discontent with the shortened curriculum has been voiced, and one has the feeling that four years will be the eventual compromise. There has also been a recent tightening of testing procedures and a greater emphasis on teaching basics, both of which became slipshod following the Cultural Revolution.

There are five faculties of stomatology in China, all associated with medical colleges: Peking Medical College, Shanghai Second Medical College, Szechwan Medical College, Hangkow-Hupei Provincial Medical College, and Chung King Fourth Military Medical College. The last-named faculty produces dental personnel for the Peoples Liberation Army.

Dental colleges seem to be well endowed with faculty. At Peking, for example, sixty faculty were teaching 180 students—three classes of 60 each. Other schools appear to have from 96 to 120 students in each of three classes. This ratio contrasts sharply to that in medicine; Cheng and Axelrod believe there are one hundred medical colleges in China and 150,000 students of medicine, 50,000 in each entering class.[1]

All told, there may be about 1,500 students of stomatology in China, with 500 entering and graduating each year. This figure represents more graphically than any other the low priority the Chinese Ministry of Health places on advanced dental treatment. If it were not for the reconstituted village tooth pullers and acupuncturists and the lesser trained dental technicians, most Chinese people would receive no dental care.

Students in dentistry are selected by the same method as those in medicine: having been recommended by their fellow workers and their commune revolutionary committee, they apply, sit for an examination, are reviewed by the faculty of stomatology and, finally, are selected by the university revolutionary committee. Before entering the three year curriculum, professional students all take a six month "cultural reading" course designed to bring them up to speed in basic sciences.

The first year of college is basic science, taken with the medical students. In addition, some basic dental technique courses are taught. The second year offers general medical courses, ward rounds, and so forth, as well as dental clinical exposure. The third year is devoted to clinical stomatology. One must remember, however, that about one-third of a student's time is spent on a commune or at a collective, where he works with the peasants in groups of ten students and five faculty. Part of this time, of course, he may be working with the commune dental workers.

After graduation (they receive no degree, but nonetheless are called "doctor," as are even barefoot doctors), the young dentist serves for at least two years in a clinical capacity. The best of the lot are then tapped to go into administration or to return for specialty training. Political considerations may play some role in these decisions. Some of the specialists continue training for as long as two or three years.

It would appear that about a third of the stomatologists working or training in China are women.

INCIDENCE OF DENTAL DISEASE IN CHINA

To the untrained eye, the Chinese appear to have "great teeth." Upon closer examination, however, one notices a high incidence of periodontal disease in adults and a good many missing posterior teeth. Older Chinese proudly exhibit anterior gold crowns. Only stainless crowns are used today, some open-faced, some with plastic facings.

There is absolutely no information out of China concerning the prevalence of dental disease or the results of treatment. Only two examinations have been reported by Western dentists.

In 1975, Dr. Reginald Louie, of the U.S. Public Health Service, had the opportunity to examine thirty-two children at the Yen-Dun Street Kindergarten in Kwangchou (Canton) and ten children (five and a half to six years) at a factory-based kindergarten at the Peking No. 3 cotton mill. He reports that

the children examined in Kwangchou ranged in age from three-and-a-half to six-and-a-half years and had an average def rate of 2.72 and gingival debris index of 1.56 (scale 0—4 low to high). Many of these children had very severe caries and moderate gingival debris, as did several of the children in Peking.[2]

In spite of the decayed and missing rate in some of the children, half of them (sixteen) had a def rate of 1.0 or less (see Table 18–3).

In 1973, I had the opportunity to examine casually thirty-two seven year old children in a Shanghai school. My impression was that over half had severe caries, a number with alveolar abscesses. Many were rapidly developing gingivitis from their poor oral hygiene. None of the permanent first molars or incisors appeared to be decayed, however. My findings appear to parallel those of Louie.

At the same Shanghai school complex, I was also able to examine forty-nine fourteen year olds, eighteen girls and thirty-one boys. The contrast between these youngsters, with permanent teeth, and the young children in the first grade was startling. The fourteen year olds had virtually no caries. The only missing teeth (there were a few remaining primary teeth) were congenitally missing or premolars extracted because of *dens evaginatus*, of which there is a 2.2 percent incidence reported in orientals generally.[3] The incidence of gingival debris and caries was only slightly less in the fourteen year old girls than in the boys (see Table 18–4).

Mild gingivitis forecast the future periodontal problems apparent in adult Chinese. Since Shanghai does not fluoridate its water supply, mottling of some of the teeth of the fourteen year olds might indicate the presence of natural fluorine in the water supplies. Each child had been born in Shanghai, most within the First Shanghai Workers' Village where the schools were located. Mottling was not found in the first grade children. Kwangchou is apparently the only Chinese city with part of its water supply fluoridated.

The wide disparity in caries incidence between primary and permanent teeth in Chinese children calls for some explanation. Louie[4] points out that there appears to be a

> widely marketed packaged mix that contains powdered milk, sugar and other ingredients. Many parents feed this solution, using milk bottles, to [their] young; it is frequently given as an adjunct to sleep. This practice is particularly interesting since breast feeding is so widely encouraged and practiced by 90–95 percent of mothers in the urban areas until the infant is about 12 months, and in the rural areas until 18 months. In any event, this practice may have a direct causal relationship to the high rate of caries in the young children examined.

This glaring difference between primary and permanent teeth has been noted in other oriental populations as well, and the explanation remains obscure.

Table 18—3. Yen-Dun Street Kindergarten— Kwangchou, PRC.

Age	Permanent Tooth Caries DEF	Gingival (Debris)	Remarks [Louie]
Females			
1. 3-1/2	6D 2F	1	
2. "	7	1	
3. "	0	1	
4. "	4 (upper incisor decayed to gumline)	1	
5. "	0	2	
6. "	1	1	
7. 4-1/2	1 (upper central incisor)	1	
8. 5-1/3	7 (mostly anterior interproximal)	2	
9. "	8	1	
10. "	4	1	
11. "	4	0	
12. "	3 (upper incisors)	3	
13. 6	4	2	
14. "	7	3	
15. "	1	3	
16. "	0	1	
17. "	0	2	
18. "	6	1	
19. "	2	1	
20. "	0	2	
21. "	1	3	
22. "	0	2	

Males				
1.	3-1/2	4 (anterior mottling)	0	
2.	"	0	2	
3.	"	2 (upper central incisors)	1	Missing 2 lower incisors
4.	"	0	3	
5.	5-1/3	0	0	
6.	"	1	1	
7.	"	6	2	
8.	6.	1	2	
9.	"	0	1	
10.	6-1/2	5D (5 deciduous molars missing)	3	All 6 year molars and all centrals erupted; missing, all upper deciduous incisors

Table 18-4. Dental Examination of Forty-nine Children—Fourteen Years of Age in Middle School—First Shanghai Workers' Village, Eighteen Girls and Thirty-one Boys.

Number	Caries	Gingival	Comments	[Ingle]
Females				
1	0	+1		
2	0	0		
3	0	0		
4	+0.5	0		
5	0	0		
6	0	0.5		
7	+1	+1	hypoplasia	
8	0	0		
9	0	0		
10	0	0	hypoplasia	
11	0	0	mottling, mild	
12	+0.5	+1	2 missing, lower premolars	
13	0	0		
14	0	+1		
15	0	+0.5		
16	0	+2		
17	0	+0.5		
18	+1	+2		
Average	0.16	0.53	Scale: 0 to +4	
Males				
1	+1	+1		
2	0	+1		
3	0	+1	deciduous teeth remaining	
4	0	+1	mottling, mild	
5	0	0	mottling, mild	
6	0	0	mottling, mild	
7	0	0		
8	0	+1	#7 missing, #10 peg-shaped	
9	0	0		
10	+1	+1	1 amalgam	
11	0	+1	severely malposed	
12	0	+2		
13	0	+1	mottling, mild	
14	0	+2	unerupted teeth	
15	0	+2	mottling, mild	
16	0	0		
17	0	0	hypoplasia	
18	+0.5	+2		
19	0	0	mottling, mild	
20	0	+0.5	mottling, mild	
21	0	+1	mottling, mild	
22	+0.5	0	mottling, mild	
23	0	+0.5		
24	0	+0.5		
25	0	0		
26	0	+1	malposed	

Table 18–4. continued.

Number	Caries	Gingival	Comments	[Ingle]
Males (cont.)				
27	0	+0.5	deciduous teeth remaining	
28	+1	+1	hypoplasia and 1 amalgam	
29	0	+0.5	mottling, mild	
30	0	+2	heavy calculus, 23–26	
31	0	0	wide spacing	
Average	0.13	0.77	Scale: 0 to +4	

CONCLUSIONS

All in all, China has not met her potential in dentistry, either in care or prevention—particularly in the latter. But then, what country has? Dentistry evidently does not have a high priority in the master plans of the Ministry of Health.

A good deal of attention in China is directed to applying traditional Chinese treatments—acupuncture, herbal concoctions, and so forth—to dentistry.[5] In no way, however, is this a substitute for the impact a well thought out and well carried out prevention program would have.

With the rigid controls and the unbelievable cooperation that are the norm among Chinese people, it stands to reason that a very effective dental prevention program could be mounted and carried out in the school systems. That they have not seen fit to undertake a massive program in prevention probably reflects the low priority the Chinese people seem to place on retaining their teeth.

China has unquestionably chosen the proper course in the delivery of dental care, however. The government has learned that there is no need to pay someone 200 yuan a month to carry out uncomplicated dental procedures when someone can be trained in a fraction of the time and paid 50 yuan to do the same thing just as well. Sophisticated Chinese practitioners are saved for sophisticated procedures, as well as for management. This may be the lesson some of the other developing nations could learn from China.

NOTES

1. Tsung O. Cheng, Lloyd Axelrod, and Alexander Leaf, Medical Education and Practice in People's Republic of China, *Ann Int. Med.* 83 (November 1975): 716–24.

2. Reginald Louie, Dental Care in the People's Republic of China (in press, June 1977).

3. John I. Ingle, *Endodontics*, 2nd ed. (Philadelphia: Lea & Febiger, 1976), pp. 316–18.

4. Louie.

5. Ingle, pp. 523–24.

ABOUT THE AUTHOR

Dr. Ingle is senior professional associate at the Institute of Medicine, National Academy of Sciences, Washington, D.C. In 1973, as a member of a medical mission from the IOM, Dr. Ingle visited Mainland China as a guest of the Chinese Medical Association. As the only dentist with the mission, he was afforded an unusual opportunity to observe the Chinese dental as well as medical systems.

Prior to joining the staff of the institute, Dr. Ingle was dean of the School of Dentistry at the University of Southern California. Before moving to Los Angeles, he served for sixteen years on the dental faculty at the University of Washington in Seattle.

Dr. Ingle received his D.D.S. degree from Northwestern University in 1942 and his Master's degree (periodontology) from the University of Michigan in 1948.

His present address is: Institute of Medicine, 2101 Constitution Avenue, Washington, D.C. 20418.

Chapter 19

Dental Care Delivery in the United States

Dr. Max H. Schoen

Area: 9,362,900 square kilometers
Population: 218,000,000
Per Capita Gross National Product: $7,340 (1976)
Life Expectancy: seventy-one years

Diversity is characteristic of dentistry, as it is for all aspects of life in the United States. In consequence, any summary such as this one is oversimplified, because it necessarily emphasizes means, medians, and dominant modes. The problem of giving a true picture of American dentistry is further complicated by the woeful inadequacy of research into dental health in the United States. Many of the relevant studies, sometimes the only studies that deal with certain subjects, are more than a decade old—unfortunate in a setting of rapid change. Despite these problems, this chapter will attempt to outline the results of whatever research has been done and to raise some of the issues that are implicit in the dental delivery system we have today.

DENTAL PERSONNEL

Dentists

In 1975, there were about 125,000 dentists in the United States, about 80 percent of them in independent practice, for a ratio of forty-seven practicing independent dentists per 100,000 population (1:2,130). But geographical distribution is very uneven (Table 19–1). Thus, ratios by state in 1976 ranged from seventy-seven per 100,000 (1:1,300) in New York to twenty-nine per 100,000 (1:3,450) in Mississippi.[1] In 1972, there were over 550 counties, containing a total of

Table 19–1.   Distribution of U.S. Dentists and Population by Region, 1976.

Region	Number of Dentists	Estimated Population	Dentists per 100,000	Dentist to Population
New England	7,997	12,198,000	66	1:1,525
Middle Atlantic	25,207	37,263,000	68	1:1,479
South Atlantic	15,587	33,715,000	46	1:2,161
East South Central	5,162	13,544,000	38	1:2,605
East North Central	20,917	40,979,000	51	1:1,960
West North Central	9,044	16,690,000	54	1:1,854
West South Central	8,493	20,856,000	41	1:2,454
Mountain	5,216	9,645,000	54	1:1,855
Pacific	19,194	28,234,000	68	1:1,470
United States Total	124,659*	213,121,000		

*This figure includes 7,842 in the federal dental services, which are not in the regional numbers.

Source: American Dental Association, Bureau of Economic Research and Statistics, *Facts About States for the Dentist Seeking a Location—1976.* (Chicago, 1976).

Table 19–2.   Dental Specialists in the United States, 1960–1976.

	1960	1970	1976	Percent in 1976
Endodontists	–	497	640	6
Oral Pathologists	42	97	68	1
Oral Surgeons	1,183	2,406	2,937	26
Orthodontists	2,097	4,335	4,667	41
Pedodontists	229	1,159	1,256	11
Periodontists	307	1,003	1,067	9
Prosthodontists	278	715	719	6
Public Health	34	103	83	1
Total	4,170	10,315	11,437	
Percent of all dentists	4	9	9	

Sources: American Dental Association, Bureau of Economic Research and Statistics, *Facts About States for a Dentist Seeking a Location— 1976* (Chicago, 1976); and National Center for Health Statistics, U. S. Department of Health, Education, and Welfare, *Health Resources Statistics— Health Manpower and Health Facilities, 1974* (Washington, D.C: GPO, 1974).

over two and a half million persons, that had either no dentist at all or fewer than seventeen per 100,000 (1:6,000)[2]—and the situation has not improved much since.[3]

Nine percent of the dentists (more than 11,000 in 1976) were specialists. This was more than two and a half times the number of specialists in 1960, although the rate of increase appears to be leveling off (Table 19–2). The largest single specialty was orthodontics, comprising 41 percent of all specialists, followed by oral surgery at 26 percent. As in the case of all dentists, geographic distribution of specialists was very uneven, with 25 percent located in California and New York (which together have only 18 percent of the population); California alone had 16 percent of the orthodontists for 10 percent of the population.[4]

Dentistry in the United States has been the preserve of the white male. Only 2.3 percent of all dentists in 1970 were black and 1.3 percent Hispanic. Virtually none were native Americans. Only 3.4 percent were women.[5]

Auxiliary Personnel

Most auxiliaries, except laboratory technicians, are women, with the low proportions of black and Hispanics similar to those for dentists.[6]

In 1973, private practitioners employed 41,000 dental hygienists, of whom over half worked part time (Table 19—3). Almost all of the 145,000 dental assistants worked full time, as did over 80 percent of the 57,000 secretary-receptionists.[7] In 1975, most dentists employed a dental assistant, but about 35 percent had no secretary-receptionist and almost 60 percent had no hygienist (Table 19—4). Most of the dental laboratory technicians work in an extensive network of commercial laboratories around the country. (On average, dentists spent only two and a half hours per week in the laboratory.)[8]

Paradental personnel similar to New Zealand dental nurses or to denturists, as recently licensed in Canada, are not legal in the United States. However, starting with Iowa in 1969, a few states have liberalized their dental practice acts to permit assistants and/or hygienists to perform such duties as placing and polishing composite and amal-

Table 19—3. Estimated Number of Auxiliary Personnel Employed by Independent Dentists in the United States, 1973.

Type	Number of Employees		
	Full Time	Part Time	Total
Hygienists	19,700	21,300	41,000
Technicians	4,800	2,500	7,300
Assistants	115,800	28,900	144,700
Secretary-Receptionist	46,700	10,400	57,100
Total	187,000	63,100	250,100

Source: American Dental Association, Bureau of Economic Research and Statistics *The 1973 Survey of Dental Practice* (Chicago: American Dental Association, 1974).

Table 19—4.   Dental Auxiliaries in the United States, 1975.

	None (percent)	One Full Time (percent)	Two or More Full Time (percent)	Median Monthly Salary
Hygienists	58.7	18.6	3.3	$810.00
Chairside Assistants	7.5	52.0	35.7	500.00
Secretaries	35.8	49.5	8.7	522.00

Source: American Dental Association, Bureau of Economic Research and Statistics, *The 1975 Survey of Dental Practice* (Chicago, 1977).

gam restorations or, in the case of hygienists, injecting local anesthetics. Dentists must prepare all cavities, however. By 1973, forty-four states permitted some form of expanded function, though both legislation and implementation vary considerably from state to state and constant changes are occurring.[9]

Specific information as to how many dentists are actually using auxiliaries in expanded capacities is not available. However, in 1975, 16 percent of independent dentists employed more than three full-time auxiliaries, and it seems reasonable to assume that many of these performed expanded functions, lawful or not.[10]

MODE OF PRACTICE

The predominant mode of practice in the United States is private, solo, fee for service. In 1975, about two-thirds of all independent dentists practiced without any business arrangements with other dentists, and many of the others had only very loose or minor connections. The concept of large-scale group practice seems to be growing slowly, however. A 1970 survey by the Public Health Service, using a fairly structured definition of "group," identified 715 such private practices, involving 3,148 dentists; while 10 percent had existed before 1950, the greatest growth occurred after 1965.[11]

Certain other approaches to practice deserve mention, since their importance for the future may outweigh their current size. For example, the armed forces employed 6,141 dentists in 1976, a figure that expands and contracts as the size of the armed services changes.

The Veterans Administration, in addition to providing funds to private dentists for dental care to eligible veterans, employed 777 dentists in 1975. Facilities were located in 171 hospitals, ten satellites, and six outpatient clinics.[12] Eligibility requirements for dental care are much more stringent than for general medical and hospital care. Nevertheless, this large system either provided or paid for over $100,000,000 worth of dentistry.[13]

Many of the 786 dentists employed by the United States Public Health Service in 1976[14] were engaged in research and administrative duties related to the expenditure of federal funds. But the service is also responsible for a number of programs that provide direct dental services. Two of the most interesting are the Indian Health Service and the National Health Service Corps.

The Indian Health Service, employing about 200 dentists supplemented by about 700 contracting private practitioners, is responsible for the care of over 500,000 American Indians and Alaska native people. Facilities include 147 fixed clinics, thirty mobile units, and additional portable field equipment to service almost 400 different sites. The program is also responsible for training both conventional and expanded duty auxiliaries, most of whom are from the target population.[15]

Under the National Health Service Corps, federal funding is available to pay the salaries of dentists assigned to identified shortage areas, provided that the specific communities establish nonprofit organizations to sponsor the practices. Fees collected are used to pay for facilities, auxiliaries, and other overhead expenses. As of March 1977, 714 shortage areas (45 percent in the Southeast) had been identified and ninety-eight dentists placed. Funds are available, and there are enough dentist applicants to place about twice as many, but the necessary community organizations have not been established. Most dentists are meeting a commitment to serve a limited number of years in return for a federal educational scholarship. Since the program has only been in operation since 1972, it is too early to tell how successful it will be in retaining dentists in practice in the shortage areas. To date, several have elected to stay in the corps an extra year, and fourteen have made the transition to private practice in their specific locations.[16]

Dentistry is included in the minimum package of primary care services that must be provided by law by community health centers. There are 157 such centers, mainly in urban areas; they are subsidized by the Bureau of Community Health Services of the Department of Health, Education, and Welfare and are governed by representatives of the local patient population. The level of dental coverage varies considerably from center to center.[17]

In addition, nonfederal government bodies conduct numerous dental care programs with differing coverages and services. Most of these are directed toward children or at least have them as a special priority. The exact number of persons affected is not known. One example of an effective, efficient program is that of the Philadelphia Department of Public Health, under which children are treated in health centers by dentists utilizing expanded duty dental assistants or technotherapists. When this system was substituted for the more traditional mode, productivity per dentist was quadrupled while costs only doubled.[18]

About half the population of the United States is covered by fluoridated water systems, and a variety of public and semipublic programs are in operation. Many of these are study and demonstration projects. A recent analysis of the results of programs whose primary goal is health education has raised serious questions as to their efficacy and efficiency.[19]

DENTAL EDUCATION

In order to qualify for the licensure necessary for practice in each state, dentists and hygienists must have graduated from an accredited dental school. In 1976, there were fifty-nine such schools and one more in the planning stage. All were university-based, and thirty-five were attached to state universities. Within recent years, a new category of private university dental school has emerged, a quasi-private school that receives some state aid. By 1977, eleven schools were in this category whereas thirteen schools were still considered private (Table 19—5).

Dentists

Dental curricula are usually four years long, although several schools experimented with an intense three year program for a time.[20] Dental schools also provide advanced specialty education, but most general practice residencies are at other institutions, primarily hospitals.[21]

The increase in both number and size of dental schools has been stimulated in large measure by federal government funding and its associated requirements. All schools, whether public or private, received support from federal and/or state sources.[22] Besides con-

Table 19—5. Status of U.S. Dental Schools, 1976—1977.

Dental Schools	Number
Public	35
Private	13
Private—State	11
	59

Source: American Dental Association, Council on Dental Education, Division of Educational Measurements, *Annual Report 1976/77* (Chicago, 1976).

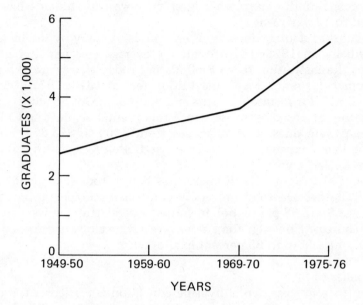

Figure 19–1. U.S. Dental School Graduates, 1950–1976. *(Graduating class has grown from 2,565 to 5,336. Sharp upturn in 1970 relates to Health Professions Assistance Act.)*

Source: American Dental Association Council on Dental Education, Division of Educational Measurements, *1976 Annual Report on Dental Education* (Chicago, 1976); also, National Center for Health Statistics, DHEW, *Health Resources Statistics—Health Manpower and Health Facilities, 1974.* (Washington, D.C.: GPO, 1974).

tinuing support for schools, the latest federal Health Professionals Assistance Act provides for optional offsite clinical teaching in ambulatory care settings. Additional provisions are designed to encourage training for primary care and multiple auxiliary team practice.[23]

Over 80 percent of entering dental students have bachelor's degrees. In 1976, there were 5,336 dental graduates, more than double the number in 1950 (Figure 19–1). As recently as 1970, there were only 3,749 graduates.[24] This large increase, coupled with the falling birth rate, is reversing postwar trends in dentist to population ratios. Minority enrollment in dental schools is considerably greater than the existing proportion of minority dentists, though it is growing only slowly. For example, 1976–1977 minority graduates were 4 percent black, 0.9 percent Mexican-American, and 0.1 percent American Indian, compared to a first year enrollment of 4.9, 1.4, and 0.3 percent, respectively. Women dental students, on the other hand, are increasing rapidly. Current expected women graduates are

7.6 percent of the class, while first year women students have increased to 13.5 percent.[25]

The cost of dental education is enormous. A study by the Institute of Medicine in 1972–1973 found the average cost per student per year to the institution to be $9,050, and today's costs are undoubtedly much higher.[26] First year tuition fees in 1976–1977 averaged only $2,615 for instate residents and $3,498 for out of staters—only a fraction of actual expenses—in public dental schools and higher still in private ones. Tuition ranges from $300 to $13,875, not including living expenses or instrument and other fees, which can be as high as $2,186 a year.[27]

Financial support for students has come from scholarships and loans. The average total university-controlled scholarship money in 1975 was $95,268 per school, including federal, state, university, and other sources. However, the students receiving aid varied from 6 percent in one school to 95 percent in another.[28]

Auxiliaries

Two to four year dental hygiene education is carried out at community colleges and dental schools. Between 1965 and 1974, the annual number of graduates increased from 1,492 to 4,313, due largely to the expansion of community college programs.[29]

Even though dental assistants and dental laboratory technicians are not required to have formal training, the number completing such education at community colleges has increased dramatically in recent years. Graduating assistants increased from 1,241 in 1965 to 5,684 in 1974, while lab technicians went from 119 to 839 over the same period (Figure 19–2). In the ten years between 1965 and 1974, the ratio of all auxiliaries to dentists climbed from 0.9 to 2.4 auxiliaries for every dentist (Figure 19–3).[30] As expanded function regulations are implemented, there will probably be increasing emphasis on formal education at approved institutions for dental assistants.

TEAM (Training in Expanded Auxiliary Management) programs for dental students have allowed dental schools to train their own expanded duty auxiliaries, since such courses were not available elsewhere. Similarly, programs such as the Indian Health Service and the one conducted by the Philadelphia Department of Health have done their own training, although some continuing education programs are beginning to include such courses.

Continuing Education

Short courses enabling dentists to maintain and improve their skills are widely available. They are usually sponsored by dental

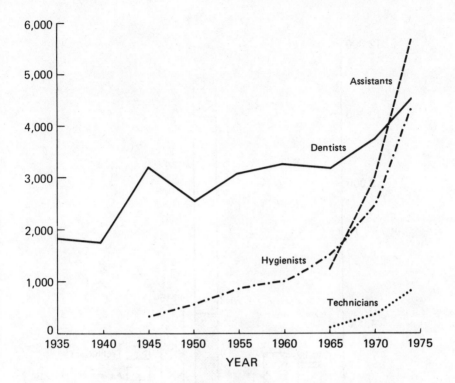

Figure 19-2. Number of U.S. Dentist and Dental Auxiliary Graduates at Selected Five Year Intervals, Through 1974.

Source: DHEW, Health Resources Administration, Division of Dentistry, *Dentist and Dental Auxiliary Graduates,* by State and Individual Institution, DHEW Publication No. HRA 77-7, (Washington, D.C.: U.S. Government Printing Office, 1977).

schools and universities, but dental societies, hospitals, and other institutions also offer them. Continuing education courses are available for dental ancillaries, but in far fewer numbers. Several states (for example, California) now require evidence of such education for maintenance of licensure.

Outreach Programs

One aspect of dental education that might almost be considered a mode of practice is the dental school outreach program. There are a number of these throughout the country, and they utilize either fixed, mobile, or portable facilities, often in cooperation with grassroots community organizations. One highly successful program for

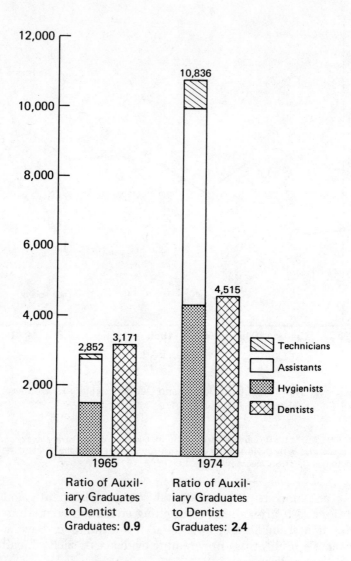

Figure 19—3.   Number of U.S. Dental Auxiliary and Dentist Graduates and Auxiliary to Dentist Graduate Ratios, 1965 and 1974.

Source: DHEW, Health Resources Administration, Division of Dentistry, *Dentist and Dental Auxiliary Graduates,* by State and Individual Institution, DHEW Publication No. HRA 77—7, (Washington, D.C.: U.S. Government Printing Office, 1977).

children of migrant farm laborers was started by students at the University of Southern California and is now under the guidance of the faculty. It combines the use of two mobile trailers and additional portable equipment for over twenty chairs. Each operative station costs $150; a functional cardboard dental chair, developed by students in the school of design, is in use. At present, 1,500 children are treated annually by volunteer students and faculties from USC and UCLA. The local communities supply meals and lodging, county government provides supplies, and there is some federal funding under a program for migrant workers.[31]

DENTAL CARE FINANCING

In fiscal year 1976, $8.6 billion, or $39.38 per capita, was spent for dental care, compared with $940 million and $6.12 per capita in 1950 (Table 19-6).[32] During this period, dental fees increased 2.7 times, only slightly more than the general inflation of 2.4 times.[33] The much greater increase in total and per capita dental expenditures therefore represents the effects of population growth and, even more important, the delivery of a much larger amount of dental care.

Last year, private insurance paid 13 percent of dental expenses, government 5 percent, and the balance was paid out of pocket (Table 19-7). Even though dental insurance is still quite small compared with medical and hospital insurance, it is expanding rapidly. In 1962, only about one million persons were covered; in 1970, there were twelve million; and in 1974, over thirty-three million—15 percent of the population.[34]

Most coverage is through employee or employer-sponsored group arrangements with commercial insurance companies, dental service corporations, Blue Cross, Blue Shield, or other independent plans, in descending order of frequency (Table 19-8).[35] Medicare covers very little dentistry, and unfortunately, fewer than half a million persons over sixty-five had other coverage in 1974.

Table 19-6. Expenditures for Dental Care in the United States, 1950–1976.

Year	Total (in millions)	Per Capita
1950	$ 940	$ 6.12
1960	1,944	10.65
1970	4,473	21.56
1976	8,600	39.38

Source: R. M. Gibson and M. S. Mueller, National Health Expenditures, Fiscal Year 1976, *Social Security Bulletin* 40 (April 1977): 3–22.

Table 19–7.   Source of Payment for Dental Care in the United States, 1976.

	Total (in millions)	Per Capita	Percent
Direct Payments	$6,970	$31.92	81
Private Insurance	1,160	5.31	13
Government	469	2.15	5
Philanthropy	–	–	–
Total	$8,600	$39.38	100*

*Total does not add up exactly due to rounding of numbers.
Source: R. M. Gibson and M. S. Mueller, National Health Expenditures, Fiscal Year 1976, Social Security Bulletin 40 (April 1977): 3–22.

The general trend in dental insurance is toward more comprehensive benefits. As distinguished from most medical plans, routine diagnostic procedures and many preventive measures are covered. Copayments and deductibles are being structured to encourage primary and secondary prevention. For example, even where deductibles are involved, they are often applied only after the initial diagnostic and preventive services are performed. General restorative, periodontic, endodontic, and surgical services are covered with relatively low patient copayments, while prosthetic and orthodontic services have higher patient out of pocket percentage payments. Maximums are becoming sufficiently high to affect only a small percent of those eligible for coverage.[36] Prepaid group practice plans will be discussed under the section on dentist reimbursement.

The $469 million spent on dental care by government in 1976 consisted primarily of payments ($390 million) to private practitioners under Medicaid, a federal–state program for the poor and medically needy.[37] This is an extremely complex program that, despite certain minimum federal requirements, has different levels of coverage and benefits in each state. Dental coverage is particularly variable, since it is not a mandated benefit. It accounts for an average of only 2.7 percent of all Medicaid expenses, far less than the proportion for the general population, with a variation from nothing in Delaware to over 10 percent in Hawaii. About $118 million, or 30 percent of dental Medicaid dollars, was spent in New York and California alone.[38]

One major mandated part of the Medicaid program since 1973 has been Early and Periodic Screening, Diagnosis, and Treatment (EPSDT) for eligible children. Although dentistry is mandated in this case, implementation has been very spotty.[39] The Carter administration has proposed modification and downgrading of this portion of

Table 19—8. Enrollment and Benefit Expenditures by Type of Dental Care, United States, 1974.

Type of Plan	Enrollment (in thousands)	Percent	Expenditures (in millions)	Percent
Blue Cross—Blue Shield	3,790	11.4	53.5	6.9
Insurance Companies	16,842	50.6	332.2	42.6
Dental Service Corporations	9,500	28.5	340.0	43.7
Other Independent Plans	3,165	9.5	52.7	6.8
Total	33,297	100	778.4	100

Source: M. S. Mueller and P. A. Pire, Private Health Insurance in 1974, *Social Security Bulletin* 39 (March 1976): 3-20.

Medicaid. In addition, some disadvantaged children have received dental care under the Headstart program.

The next largest segment of government dental expenditure is for payments of $55 million to private dentists by the Veterans Administration for dental care for eligible veterans.[40]

INCOME TO PROVIDERS

In 1969, the only reported occupational groups with incomes exceeding $15,000 per year were lawyers and judges, physicians, airplane pilots, and dentists.[41] The dentist was still in the top few percent of earners in 1975.

As stated previously, most providers are private practitioners, and most of these receive their incomes through fee for service payments. In 1974, the mean gross income of independent general practitioners was $74,000 and the net was $33,000. That for specialists was considerably higher, $97,000 and $45,000, respectively. Both gross and net incomes were closely correlated with size of facility, number of operatories, and the size of the auxiliary staff. There was surprisingly little variation by region of the country for net income, but a much greater variation for gross income, reflecting a considerable difference in operating expenses. The ages forty to fifty-four represented the peak earning years.[42]

There is some evidence that increases in productivity that have occurred over the past few decades, whether from technological innovations or increased and changed use of auxiliaries, have been primarily of financial gain to the dentists, although they have also increased the amount of dental care provided.[43]

Third parties have exercised some control of dental fees by utilizing one of three payment methods—usual, customary, and reasonable (UCR); table of allowances (T of A); and fixed fee. The T of A approach limits liability to the third party, while the other two protect both the patient and the funding source. The UCR method is preferred by organized dentistry as being more flexible, but at least one study has yielded ambiguous results as to dentists' desires.[44] Fixed fees control costs most of all but may result in underpayment for services, particularly since levels are not usually changed to keep pace with increases in the cost of living.

One major variant to fee for service is prepaid or capitation reimbursement, usually to group practices. In this case, the dental organization receives a regular periodic payment based on an enrolled population. In return, it agrees to provide a given spectrum of benefits.

Projections are based on assumptions of the quantity of resources required to provide the services and the cost of these resources.[45] The more general form of this approach is the Health Maintenance Organization.

DENTAL SERVICES AND
ORAL HEALTH STATUS

Up to this point this chapter has provided a brief overview of most aspects of dentistry in the United States, except what happens to the population. Is the American system successful? In 1974, almost half (49.3 percent) of the population saw a dentist at least once. The seventeen to twenty-four year age group had the best record, with 57.5 percent. Almost 31 percent of those under seventeen had never seen a dentist. The average number of annual visits was 1.7 per person, with very little variation,by age.[46]

Studies, as yet unpublished, from 1975, provide more detail by demographic characteristics:[47]

- For example, 35 percent of persons with incomes under $5,000 had visited the dentist within one year, compared to 65 percent for those with incomes over $15,000. Similarly, "never users" decreased from 13 percent for the low income group to 6 percent for the high income group (Table 19−9).
- The greater the amount of education, the greater the number of visits per year, regardless of age (Table 19−10a).
- Whites visited the dentist more during the year (1.7 visits) than nonwhites (1 visit), and this difference applied to all ages (Table 19−10b).
- However, the average number of visits per person per year remained virtually unchanged, with 1.5 in 1957−1958 and only 1.6 almost eighteen years later.[48]

Figures on the number of visits can be misleading, as a study conducted by the Center for Health Administration Studies found in 1964.[49] According to these data, only 1.8 percent of the population consumed 25 percent of the visits, and 18 percent, 75 percent of the visits (Figure 19−4). Only 0.8 percent of the population had 25 percent of the expenditures, and 10 percent had 75 percent of all expenditures (Figure 19−5). The higher socioeconomic groups had more expenditures, more visits, and more visits for every type of service except extractions.

Table 19—9. Number and Percent of Persons by Time Interval Since Their Last Dental Visit, by Income, United States, 1975.

	Number in Thousands		*Time Interval Since Last Visit*		
a) *Income*		*Total Population*	*Under 1 Year*	*5+ Years*	*Never*
Total		209,065	105,219	28,837	20,823
under $3,000		14,676	5,080	4,019	1,910
3,000– 4,999		17,074	5,917	4,320	2,289
5,000– 6,999		19,602	7,381	3,862	2,713
7,000– 9,999		25,671	10,977	3,939	3,174
10,000–14,999		47,103	23,628	5,345	5,309
$15,000 +		69,868	45,458	4,808	4,069
b) *Percent*					
Total		100	50	14	10
under $3,000		7	35	27	13
3,000– 4,999		8	35	25	13
5,000– 6,999		9	38	20	14
7,000– 9,999		12	37	15	12
10,000–14,999		23	50	11	11
$15,000 +		33	65	7	6

Source: Condensation of unpublished data from the Health Interview Survey, National Center for Health Statistics. (Data are based on household interviews of the civilian non-institutional population. Average totals include those with unknown income and unknown visits.)

Caries and Tooth Loss

One ultimate indicator of the effectiveness of dental care is the degree of edentulism, or tooth loss, in a population. In 1957–1958, 13 percent of the population were edentulous. This had dropped to 11.2 percent by 1971.[50] The improvement had occurred in each age group, but between 9 and 10 percent of thirty-five to forty-four year olds were still edentulous. The higher the socioeconomic status, the less the level of edentulism. For persons in the forty-five to sixty-four age bracket, the range in 1971 was between almost 37 percent for low income persons with little education to 12 percent for wealthier, more educated persons. For those sixty-five and over, the range was from 60 percent to 30 percent, respectively (Table 19—11). Of the estimated twenty-three million edentulous persons, almost two million had incomplete or no replacements, another two and a half million did not wear them all the time, and about six and a half million (30 percent) thought they were unsatisfactory.

A more recent study by the American Dental Association of wearers of prosthetic appliances estimated that there were about twenty-three and a half million totally edentulous persons in 1975.[51] Almost

Table 19-10. Number of Dental Visits per Person, per Year, by Education of the Head of the Household and by Age and Color, United States, 1975.

(a) *Education*

Age	*Under 9 Years*	*9-11 Years*	*12 Years*	*13-15 Years*	*16+ Years*
All ages	1.0	1.3	1.6	2.1	2.5
Under 17 years	1.2	1.2	1.5	1.9	2.4
17-24 years	1.1	1.7	1.8	2.3	2.3
25-44 years	0.8	1.3	1.5	2.1	2.4
45-64 years	1.1	1.4	1.8	2.3	3.0
65+ years	0.8	1.2	1.3	1.4	2.5

(b) *Color*

Age	*All Persons*	*White*	*All Others*
All ages	1.6	1.7	1.0
Under 17 years	1.6	1.7	0.8
17-24 years	1.8	1.9	1.1
25-44 years	1.7	1.7	1.2
45-64 years	1.8	1.8	1.3
65+ years	1.2	1.2	0.6

Source: Unpublished data from the Health Interview Survey, National Center for Health Statistics. (Data are based on household interviews of the civilian non-institutional population.)

twenty-six million wore at least one full denture, about sixteen and a half million wore at least one partial denture, and slightly more than five million had one or more fixed bridges. There were the expected major variations by age and socioeconomic status. Only 5 percent of those earning $20,000 or more had full dentures, and an even smaller percentage of college graduates were so afflicted. Partial denture wearers did not change much, except by age, but the higher the socioeconomic status, the higher the percentage of fixed bridge wearers.

DMF (decayed, missing, and filled permanent teeth) rates rise with income and education, possibly as an aberration of treatment, which would tend to increase the total scores. For example, young children ages six to eleven in 1963-1965 had a national average of 1.4 DMF, but the higher the income and the greater the number of years of schooling of the head of the household, the less the decayed and missing components were and the greater the filled compo-

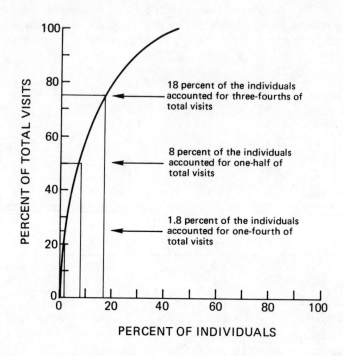

Figure 19—4. Distribution of Visits for Dental Care among U.S. Individuals, 1964.

Source: J.E. Newman and O.W. Anderson, *Patterns of Dental Service Utilization in the United States: A nationwide Social Survey* (Chicago: Center for Health Administration Studies, University of Chicago, 1972).

nent. The same differentials exist for def (primary tooth measurement).[52]

For youths ages twelve to seventeen in 1966—1970, the same general patterns prevail, although total scores are much higher, due to the annual increments of caries. For example, differences in rates between low income and high income families were 2.7 D to 0.8 D, 1.2 M to 0.2 M, and 1.6 F to 5.4 F (Figure 19—6).[53] Blacks had lower DMF rates, but the D and M components were higher and the F component much lower (Figure 19—7).

DMF continues to rise with age and in adults reflects the outcome of destructive periodontal disease and other factors as well as caries. It is sad that, for virtually all adult age categories, the D and M components exceed the F component, even with the totally edentulous excluded. Once more, the expected socioeconomic patterns prevail, with the largest differences in the filled rates.[54] For all ages, DMF is higher for whites and females (Figure 19—8).

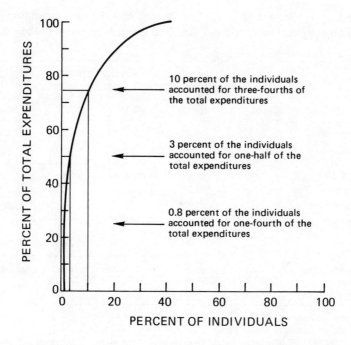

Figure 19–5. Distribution of Expenditures for Dental Care among U.S. Individuals, 1964.

Source: J.E. Newman and O.W. Anderson, *Patterns of Dental Service Utilization in the United States: A Nationwide Social Survey* (Chicago: Center for Health Administration Studies, University of Chicago, 1972).

Periodontal Disease

Using the Russell Periodontal Index as a measurement, the National Health Survey in 1960–1962 found three-fourths of the dentulous adult population with some periodontal disease and one-fourth with destructive disease.[55] Blacks and men had both more and more severe disease. Both prevalence and severity had an inverse association with income and education. There was, of course, a direct age correlation.

The same early survey suggested that about 40 percent of the dentulous adult population needed a dental visit "at an early date." Males, blacks, persons with lower incomes, and those with less education had a greater than average need, although 20–24 percent of those with high income and education also had such immediate needs.[56]

Table 19-11.   Percent of Edentulous Persons Aged Forty-five and over in United States, by Family Income, Age, and Educational Level of Individual, 1971.

Age and Educational Level	Family Income			
	All Incomes*	Less Than $5,000	$5,000– $9,999	$10,000 or more
45–64 years	Percent			
Total**	23.3	32.9	27.7	16.3
Less than 9 years	34.3	36.9	34.3	30.1
9–11 years	28.7	33.9	30.4	24.9
12 years or more	15.9	25.2	21.4	12.1
65 years and over				
Total**	50.7	56.4	46.6	38.9
Less than 9 years	58.0	60.2	56.1	50.1
9–11 years	51.1	54.9	47.0	42.4
12 years or more	37.2	46.1	33.9	29.6

*Includes unknown income.
**Includes unknown education.
Source: DHEW, National Center for Health Statistics, *Edentulous Persons— United States, 1971* (Washington, D.C.: Series 10, No. 89, U.S. Government Printing Office, 1974).

Malignancies

One projection estimated that approximately 23,800 new cases of oral cancer would occur in the United States in 1976 and that there would be 8,300 deaths. Far more men than women are affected. There appears to be more oral malignancy in lower socioeconomic groups.[57] Primary prevention is difficult and the role of dental care obscure, although a properly restored and maintained dentition should reduce some of the causative factors. However, the dentist ought definitely to be responsible for early detection and referral for treatment, with consequent decrease in massive disfigurement and mortality.

CURRENT ISSUES

A number of unresolved questions are of major concern to the dental profession, government, and the public today. This chapter can only briefly discuss a few of them.

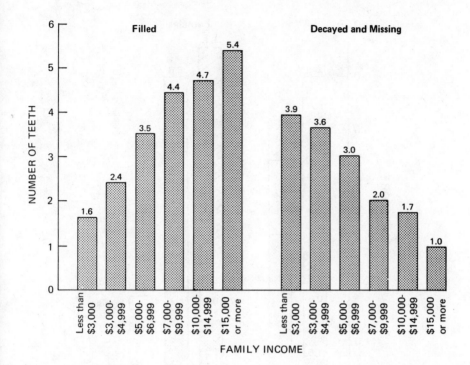

Figure 19—6. Average Number of Filled, Decayed, and Missing Permanent Teeth per Person among Youths, Twelve to Seventeen Years, by Family Income, United States, 1966—1970.

Source: National Center for Health Statistics, DHEW, *Decayed, Missing and Filled Teeth among Youth 12—17 Years, United States,* Series 11, No. 144 (Washington, D.C.: GPO, 1974).

Paradental Personnel

At present, organized dentistry has taken a position against the use of expanded function auxiliaries. A major part of the opposition is based on the capacity of dentists to treat more patients than they currently do. In 1975, over 22 percent of all independent dentists stated that they were not busy. This was about 35 percent in the Pacific region and 37 percent for orthodontists.[58]

Even if dentists are not busy and can absorb any conceivable increased demand for care, the major questions of efficiency and effectiveness are not answered. Perhaps there should be fewer dentists graduated, with consequent reallocation of tasks as ratios of different personnel arrive at more optimum levels.

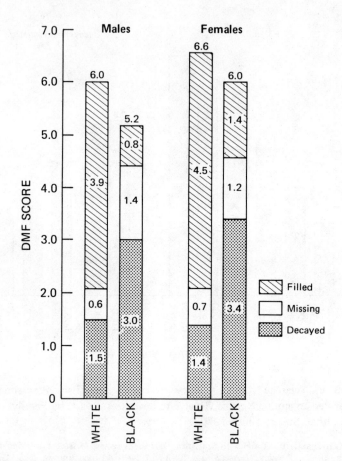

Figure 19-7. Average Number of Decayed (D), Missing (M), and Filled (F) Teeth and Average Number of DMF Components per Person among Youths, Twelve to Seventeen Years, by Sex and Race, United States, 1966–1970.

Source: National Center for Health Statistics, DHEW, *Decayed, Missing and Filled Teeth among Youth 12–17 Years, United States,* Series 11, No. 144 (Washington, D.C.: GPO, 1974).

Similar but deeper concerns exist about "dental nurses" and "denturism." If it is demonstrated that paradental personnel are as effective as dentists within their restricted areas of activity, it would appear that total opposition is a "Luddite" response. If they are not as effective, this, too, must be proved with scientific rigor. Can a lesser trained individual perform certain services as well as a dentist and, if so, under what circumstances? What will be the effect on dollar and resource costs? Serious examination, rather than unsupported

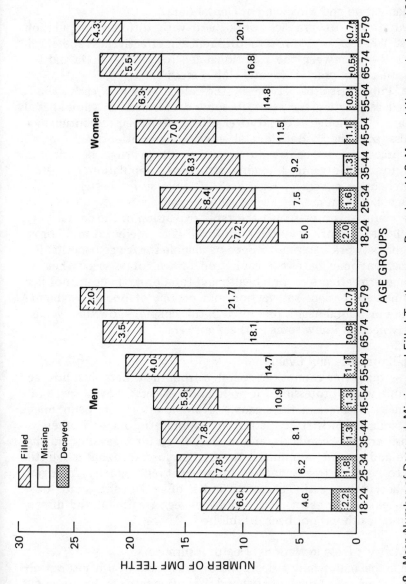

Figure 19–8. Mean Number of Decayed, Missing, and Filled Teeth among Dentulous U.S. Men and Women, by Age, 1960–1962.

Source: National Center for Health Statistics, DHEW, *Decayed, Missing and Filled Teeth in Adults. United States, 1960–1962*, Series 11, No. 23 (Washington, D.C.: GPO, 1967).

political rhetoric, must take place to protect the best interests of the public.

Organization and Financing of Dental Care

What forms of practice work best with different population groups? What, if any, long-term difference in effectiveness and efficiency is there between the traditional fee for service mode and the capitation group practice (dental HMO) mode?

The Public Health Service in the late 1940s and early 1950s achieved astounding success with some demonstration school-based programs,[59] although the carryover effect after their discontinuance was disappointing.[60] Both dental service organizations and prepaid group practices have achieved dramatic results in fringe benefit programs for well-organized, highly structured population groups.[61] Comprehensive coverage, regardless of type, seems better than no coverage, but what are the keys to the special successes?

The country is now seeing the rapid expansion of the dental "discount house," which may take the form of a "Medicaid mill" or an office or network catering to persons eligible for fringe benefits. Reimbursement may be either capitation or fee for service. What are the long-term effects on oral health and total program costs, not just on immediate patient satisfaction and on out of pocket payment? The data on dental health presented in this chapter show that we desperately need to know some of these answers.

Accountability and Evaluation

These questions cannot be separated from the others. Just how accountable is the profession for population effects? How do we evaluate these effects and their causes? Notable efforts are being made by organized dentistry,[62] institutions, administrators, and others to establish criteria, standards, and methodology for measuring quality of care and assuring a minimum level of performance, but much still needs to be done (see Schonfeld for a recent bibliography).[63] A generally acceptable, easily measured index of oral health status does not yet exist. The exact relationship between treatment and disease or dental health has not been established.

Dentistry's Role in National Health Insurance

While the major policy decisions over national health insurance—when, for whom, how administered, how financed, and so on—will be made with little relationship to dentistry, oral health does represent a special health care area requiring special treatment. Who should be covered and what benefit levels should be established? Are there sufficient resources to provide comprehensive care for all, or is a go slow, incremental approach desirable? As has been documented in this chapter, distribution of resources and their accessibility are problems, and existing approaches have barely dented the surface. But how else can this difficulty be resolved?

I have not raised issues such as licensure and reciprocity and the role of dental specialists. Some research is being conducted on the delivery questions I did raise, as well as on many of the others, but I believe it to be woefully inadequate. As has occurred so many times in the past, major policy decisions probably will be made without analyzing and taking into account current past experience. The dental profession will bear some responsibility for this state of affairs if it does not begin to organize more, and more vigorous, research into policy-related dental problems.

NOTES

1. American Dental Association, Bureau of Economic Research and Statistics, *Facts About States for the Dentist Seeking a Location—1976* (Chicago, 1976).

2. American Dental Association, Bureau of Economic Research and Statistics, *Distribution of Dentists in the United States by State, Region, District and County* (Chicago, 1964).

3 Ibid., 1974.

4. American Dental Association, *Facts About States . . . 1976.*

5. Department of HEW, Bureau of Health Resources Development, Public Health Service, Health Resources Administration, *Minorities and Women in the Health Fields*, DHEW Pub. No. (HRA) 75–22 (Washington, D.C., May 1974).

6. Ibid.

7. American Dental Association, Bureau of Economic Research and Statistics, *The 1973 Survey of Dental Practice* (Chicago, n.d.).

8. American Dental Association, Bureau of Economic Research and Statistics, *The 1975 Survey of Dental Practice* (Chicago, 1977).

9. Donald W. Johnson and Frank M. Holz, *Legal Provisions on Expanded Functions for Dental Hygienists and Assistance. Summarized by State—1973*, DHEW Pub. No. (HRA) 75–21, revised July 1974 (Washington, D.C.: U.S. Government Printing Office, 1974).

10. American Dental Association, *The 1975 Survey of Dental Practice.*

11. DHEW, Public Health Service, *Group Practice of Dentistry . . . an organizational form for the delivery of dental services*, DHEW Pub. No. (HRA) 77–8 (Washington, D.C.: Government Printing Office, 1977).

12. Marvin Marcus and Leonard Drabek, *Study: V.A. Dental Manpower Requirements* (Los Angeles: School of Dentistry, UCLA, 1976).

13. Ibid.

14. ADA, *Facts About States . . . 1976.*

15. Robert Mecklenburg, Personal communication and unpublished material, 1977.

16. Robert Beck, Personal communication, 1977.

17. Bureau of Community Health Services, Health Services Administration, Public Health Service, *Promoting Community Health—1976* (Washington, D.C.: Government Printing Office, 1976).

18. David A. Soricelli, Implementation of the Delivery of Dental Services by Auxiliaries—the Philadelphia Experience, *American Journal of Public Health* 62 (August 1972): 1077–87.

19. P. Jean Frazier, The Effectiveness and Practicability of Current Dental Health Education Programs from a Public Health Perspective: A Conceptual Appraisal (presented at the Annual Meeting of the American Public Health Association, Miami Beach, October 20, 1976).

20. American Dental Association, Council on Dental Education, Division of Educational Measurements, *1976/77 Annual Report on Dental Education* (Chicago, 1976).

21. Ibid., Advanced Dental Education Supplement.

22. Ibid.

23. DHEW, Health Resources Administration, Public Health Service, *Fact Sheet—Health Professions Educational Assistance Act of 1976* (PL 94–484) (Washington, D.C., 1976).

24. ADA, *1976/77 Annual Report*; and DHEW, Health Resources Administration, Division of Dentistry, *Dentist and Dental Auxiliary Graduates, by State and Individual Institution*, DHEW Publication No. HRA 77–7, compiled 1976 (Washington, D.C.: U.S. Government Printing Office, 1977).

25. American Dental Association, *1976/77 Annual Report.* Dental Education Supplement #3, Minority Report.

26. Institute of Medicine, *Costs of Education in the Health Professions, Report of a study*, pts. I, II, and III (Washington, D.C.: National Academy of Sciences, January 1974).

27. ADA, *1976/77 Annual Report.*

28. Ibid.

29. Ibid.; and DHEW, *Dentist and Dental Auxiliary Graduates.*

30. Ibid.

31. Charles Goldstein, Personal communication, 1977.

32. Robert M. Gibson and Marjorie Smith Mueller, National Health Expenditures, Fiscal Year 1976, *Social Security Bulletin* 40 (April 1977): 3–22.

33. Current Operating Statistics, *Social Security Bulletin* 40 (April 1977): 91–92.

34. Marjorie Smith Mueller and Paula A. Pire, Private Health Insurance in 1974. A Review of Coverage, Enrollment and Financial Experience, *Social Security Bulletin* 39 (March 1976): 3–20.

35. Ibid.

36. The Wyatt Company, *A Study of Dental Care Benefits for State Employees* (California, 1976); and Kent D. Nash, *A Study of Dental Health Related and Process Outcomes Associated with Prepaid Dental Care—Draft Research Proposal* (Research Triangle Park: Research Triangle Institute, 1977).

37. Gibson and Mueller.

38. Selvin Sonken, Personal communication including unpublished data, 1977.

39. DHEW, Medical Services Administration, Social and Rehabilitative Service, EPSDT—The Possible Dream, HEW (SRS) 77—24973 (Washington, D.C., 1977).

40. Gibson and Mueller.

41. Bureau of the Census, U.S. Department of Commerce, *Statistical Abstract of the United States—1976* (Washington, D.C.: Government Printing Office).

42. ADA, *The 1975 Survey of Dental Practice.*

43. Max M. Schoen and Neville Doherty, Dental Fees, Productivity and Income, *J. Amer. Coll. of Dent.* 41 (July 1974): 190—206; and Dale Redig, Mildred Snyder, George Nevitt, and John Tocchini, Expanded Duty Dental Auxiliaries in Four Private Dental Offices: The First Year's Experience, *JADA* 88 (May 1974): 969—48. (Also, exchange of letters between Max H. Schoen and Dale Redig, *JADA* 89 (August 1974): 238, 240.

44. Robert D. Eilers and Robert C. Jones, *The Attitudes and Anticipated Behavior of Dentists under Various Reimbursement Arrangements* (Homewood, Ill.: Irwin 1972).

45. Max M. Schoen, Methodology of Capitation Payment to Group Dental Practice and Effects of Such Payment on Care, *Health Services Reports* 89 (January-February 1974): 16—24; and Max H. Schoen, Dental Care and the Health Maintenance Organization Concept, *MMFQ* (Health and Society) 53 (Spring 1975): 173—93.

46. DHEW, National Center for Health Statistics, *Current Estimates from the Health Interview Survey. United States—1974,* DHEW Pub. No. (HRA 76—1527, Series 10, No. 100 (Washington, D.C.: Government Printing Office, September 1975).

47. DHEW, National Center for Health Statistics, Dental Visits—Time Interval Since Last Visit. United States—update to 1975 (personal communication, September 1977).

48. DHEW, National Center for Health Statistics, *Volume of Dental Visits: United States—July 1963—June 1964,* Series 10, No. 23 (Washington, D.C.: Government Printing Office, October 1965).

49. John F. Newman and Odin W. Anderson, *Patterns of Dental Service Utilization in the United States: A Nationwide Social Survey* (Chicago: Center for Health Administration Studies, University of Chicago, 1972).

50. DHEW, National Center for Health Statistics, *Edentulous Persons. United States—1971,* Series 10, No. 89 (Washington, D.C.: Government Printing Office, 1974).

51. Bureau of Economic Research and Statistics, American Dental Association, *Prosthodontic Care—Number and Type of Denture Wearers, 1975* (Chicago, 1976).

52. DHEW, Nationl Center for Health Statistics, *Decayed, Missing, and Filled Teeth Among Children. United Stated,* Series 11, No. 106 (Washington, D.C.: Government Printing Office, 1971).

53. DHEW, National Center for Health Statistics, *Decayed, Missing, and Filled Teeth Among Youths 12–17 Years. United States*, Series 11, No. 144 (Washington, D.C.: Government Printing Office, 1974).

54. DHEW, National Center for Health Statistics, *Decayed, Missing, and Filled Teeth in Adults. United States—1960–1962*, Series 11, No. 23 (Washington, D.C.: Government Printing Office, 1967).

55. DHEW, National Center for Health Statistics, *Periodontal Disease in Adults. United States—1960–1962*, Series 11, No. 12 (Washington, D.C.: Government Printing Office, 1965).

56. DHEW, National Center for Health Statistics, *Need for Dental Care Among Adults. United States—1960–1962*, Series 11, No. 36 (Washington, D.C.: Government Printing Office, 1970).

57. Theodore E. Bolden, Epidemiology of Oral Cancer (Chapter 7) and Factors Related to Oral Cancer (Cahpter 8), in Robert C. Caldwell and Richard E. Stallard, *A Textbook of Preventive Dentistry* (Philadelphia: W.B. Saunders, 1977).

58. ADA. *The 1975 Survey of Dental Practice.*

59. George E. Waterman and John W. Knutson, *Studies on Dental Care Services for School Children—Third and Fourth Treatment*, Series 69 (Richmond, Ind., Public Health Reports, March 1954) pp. 247–54; and Frank E. Law, Carl E. Johnson, and John W. Knutson, *Studies on Dental Care Services for School Children—Third and Fourth Treatment*, Series 70 (Woonsocket, R.I., Public Health Reports, April 1955), 402–409.

60. Donald J. Galagan, Frank E. Law, George E. Waterman, and Grace Scholz Spitz, Dental Health Status of Children Five Years After Completing School Care Programs, *Public Health Reports* 79 (May 1964): 445–54.

61. U.S. Public Health Service, Division of Dental Public Health and Resources, *Report on the Dental Program of the ILWU—PMA—The First Three Years*, PHS Publication No. 894 (Washington, D.C.: Government Printing Office, 1962); Max H. Schoen, Observation of Selected Dental Services under Two Prepayment Mechanisms, Dr. P.H. dissertation (Ann Arbor: University Microfioms, 1969); and Walter J. Pelton, Dental Health Program of the University of Alabama in Birmingham: IX. A Summary of Seven Years Experience, *AJPH* 62 (May 1972): 671–675.

62. California Dental Association, *Quality Evaluation for Dental Care. Guidelines for the Assessment of Clinical Quality and Professional Performance and the Standards for Program Design to Assure the Quality of Care*, Field Test Edition (Los Angeles, 1976).

63. Hyman K. Schonfeld, Evaluation of the Quality of Oral Care Systems (Chapter V), in *Oral Health, Dentistry and the American Public*, William E. Brown, ed. (Norman: University of Oklahoma Press, 1974).

ABOUT THE AUTHOR

Dr. Max Schoen is professor and chairman of preventive dentistry and public health at the University of California in Los Angeles. He also holds a joint appointment in the School of Public Health. Dr. Schoen has recently been appointed assistant dean for academic affairs at UCLA.

Before joining the UCLA faculty, Dr. Schoen was dean protem of the School of Dental Medicine at the State University of New York, Stony Brook.

Dr. Schoen is one of the pioneers in group practice in the United States, having been a founding partner and dental director of an important group practice in Los Angeles.

Dr. Schoen received both his B.S. and D.D.S. degrees from the University of Southern California and his Master's and Doctorate in public health from UCLA. He is a member of the Institute of Medicine.

His present address is: UCLA School of Dentistry, Los Angeles, California 90024.

✳   *Part VI*

New Research Findings

The ongoing International Collaborative Study here reported by Dr. Lois Cohen Now involves nearly a dozen nations. So little research has been done in international dental care delivery methods, particularly of a longitudinal nature, that this collaborative arrangement between the World Health Organization and the Division of Dentistry of the U.S. Public Health Service serves as a landmark.

One of the most significant findings to come out of the study is the perverse nature of people worldwide. It would appear that many individuals prefer being edentulous over retaining their teeth. Even those entering adulthood with all their teeth intact appear to have so little regard for their future that they are willing to submit to extractions. And what of the profession, trained to retain and maintain the dentition, who are overseeing its removal?

The ultimate answer, of course, is prevention of dental disease. As a fitting climax to this colloquium, Dr. Ahlberg describes a Swedish preventive program that could be as much a watershed as the New Zealand plan was fifty years ago.

Chapter 20

Dental Care Delivery in Seven Nations: The International Collaborative Study of Dental Manpower Systems in Relation to Oral Health Status*

Dr. Lois K. Cohen

The international collaborative study originated from the need felt by the United States Public Health Service (USPHS) and the World Health Organization (WHO) for objective data concerning the relative success of various national dental care delivery systems. USPHS wanted insights into system components that might be incorporated into plans for some type of U.S. health program. WHO wished to use the information to sharpen its consultation to countries, increasing the probability that its recommendations on public health planning would be appropriate and could be implemented. The nations that joined in the planning of the protocol, and later joined the study itself, were concerned whether their system of dental care was the most suitable for their people. Thus, the research project was designed from the start to discover which parts of a delivery system function efficiently for a given society and might also be helpful to other societies.

The specific purpose of the study is to define the relationships between structural characteristics of major national systems and selected measures of effectiveness and efficiency for the consumer, the provider, and the administrative setting in which they both operate.

*Appreciation is expressed to all the project staff at WHO headquarters in Geneva and in each of the participating countries: David Barmes, Sherwood Slater, Ingolf Moller, Mona Romer, James Duppenthaler, Peter Barnard, Fred Clements, Ulrich Keil, R. Peter Nippert, Masao Onisi, Takeo Shinohara, Peter Hunter, Peter Davis, Per Baerum, Harold Arnljot, Arthur Bonito, Charles Donelly, John Christiansen, Donald Beck, and many others who consulted, supervised, interviewed, recorded, coded, processed, and analyzed the data and in any way assisted this project toward meaningful progress.

The relationships within each prototypical system are emphasized rather than the differences between one country's system and another's. Biological and ecological influences characteristic of different parts of the world will be considered in the interpretation of results, but they are not controlled variables in the study.

Six prototype systems were initially selected, on the basis of four major criteria: degree of government or private enterprise; use or nonuse of auxiliaries; system of financing; and definition of target groups for receipt of services. All systems selected for study had been in existence for at least twenty years, which meant that a sizable proportion of adults had been exposed to the system.

The systems selected ranged from a predominantly private practice model in Australia, which has no major use of auxiliaries and is primarily fee for service, through the Federal Republic of Germany, where fee for service dental care and health care generally are subsidized by "sick" funds whose revenue comes equally from members and their employers. In Japan, there is a trend toward major use of operating auxiliaries in a mixed payment system of social insurance, government payment, and fee for service. In Norway's system, both private practice and government practice coexist for different consumer groups. New Zealand is like Norway in most respects, except that dental nurses instead of dentists provide care directly to children. Finally, Bulgaria, at the other end of this continuum, was selected because it has a predominantly government practice, with no major use of operating auxiliaries. While all possible combinations of types could not be empirically examined, this range was intended to provide data about prototypical systems as they exist around the globe.

Since 1972, when the study officially began, some changes and additions have taken place. Bulgaria withdrew from the collaboration; Poland entered and began data collection in April 1977. The Baltimore metropolitan area was selected to provide replicative data on the private sector model for the United States. Denmark and Canada began data collection in 1975 and 1977, respectively, and negotiations are continuing for the participation of Czechoslovakia and Egypt. In all, nine countries are presently part of this effort, with two more in prospect.

THE STUDY DESIGN

Presented here is a summary progress report from the seven countries that have completed data collection, though some of the data are still in various stages of analysis. The following sample areas will be covered:

>Sydney, Australia
>Hannover, Federal Republic of Germany
>Yamanashi, Japan
>Canterbury, New Zealand
>Trøndelag, Norway
>Baltimore, U.S.A.
>Aarhus, Denmark

Since the first five countries were part of the original study, these data have been subjected to more analysis than those from the United States and Denmark, which entered later.

The specific objective of the study at the outset was to provide data on system elements that are associated with varying levels of oral health. Conceptually, a set of hypotheses linked the structural characteristics (primarily descriptors of manpower arrangements) to effectiveness (primarily consumer outcomes) and efficiency (both provider- and consumer-related economic and social costs). The general hypotheses was that the more available, accessible, and acceptable the oral health care provided, the more positive is the effect on the population's oral health.

Of course, specific data indicators have been developed for many variables. It is important to note that the major outcome measures—"effects on the population"—are not measures of oral health status alone, for these could reflect differences in the natural environment (e.g., natural fluoride in the water supply, nutritional patterns, genetic characteristics) as well as in system features. Rather, the outcome (dependent) measures used in the study are expressed as a ratio of services provided to need within the population—in other words, to what extent do the dental services provided in a given society fill the oral health needs of that society? This concept—services to need or treatment to need ratio—helps to reduce variations caused by differences in disease prevalence that are not system-related.

Mediating between the structure of a system (independent variables) and the outcome variables (service-need ratios) are factors having to do with the efficiency with which a system operates. At what social and economic cost is any given ratio of service to need achieved? Thus, the monetary cost to the consumer, the provider, and the administrative components and the social cost to the society (reflected sometimes in outmigration of dental personnel, dissatisfaction with work, or irregular patterns of consumer dental visits) are viewed as qualifying data. These efficiency factors specify the condition with which any given service to need level is associated; they represent how the system processes goods, services, and people. Unfortunately, there is little space to deal with these data here; most of this presentation will focus on outcome variables—namely, treatment or service to need ratios.

The study design provided for the collection of data on a cross-sectional basis over the course of three or four months at each country site. Prior to data collection, considerable time was spent in planning, staffing, training, sampling, organizing, pretesting, and translation.

The sample drawn in each country was selected jointly by the WHO central staff in Geneva and the national team. The agreed upon criteria were that the survey region (1) be representative of the system; (2) not be the capital; and (3) contain a metropolitan and nonmetropolitan area large enough to accomplish the random sampling plan. As it worked out, except for Sydney (population nearly three million—and the Baltimore Standard Metropolitan Statistical Area (population two million), the metropolitan populations ranged from 20,000 to 500,000 and the nonmetropolitan populations ranged from slightly less than 100,000 in Norway to 600,000 in the Federal Republic of Germany.

The sample was to consist of a thousand eight to nine year olds and a thousand thirteen to fourteen year olds visited in school classrooms; a thousand thirty-five to forty-four year olds visited in homes or in a central location; one hundred from major provider groups (dentists, hygienists, dental nurses, etc.); and representative administrative officials able to give statistical and historical data on the overall system. Those aged thirteen to fourteen and thirty-five to forty-four were to be interviewed as well as examined clinically, while the eight to nine year olds were only examined. All others were interviewed or completed structured questionnaires.

PRELIMINARY FINDINGS

Children

Analysis of clinical and sociological data for the eight to nine year old sample in Sydney (Australia), Hannover (Germany), Yamanashi (Japan), Canterbury (New Zealand), and Trøndelag (Norway) was presented at the Federation Dentaire Internationale meeting in Chicago in September 1975. That presentation included consideration of the implications of sample means and data frequencies and of a stepwise regression analysis: the latter enabled us to study which factors

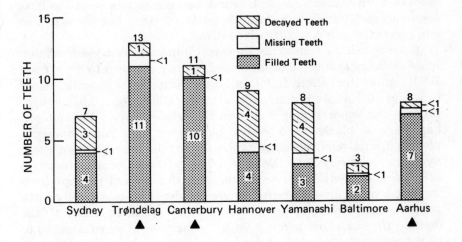

Figure 20–1. DMF Student Sample of Thirteen and Fourteen Year Olds, ICSDM Survey. *(Arrows indicate the three study sites with school-based dental care systems. Aarhus, with lowest DMF rate of three, has supported strong preventive program over ten years.)*

Source: World Health Organization—Division of Dentistry, International Collaborative Study of Dental Manpower.

were strongest in explaining variations in oral health. Both intra-country and intercountry aspects were analyzed.

The main findings highlighted the very different clinical coverage in Canterbury and Trøndelag, where structured school services are available, and that in the remaining three countries, where, in the main, restorative services were available only on demand. In the systems having school-based services, more of the need was being met than in the other systems, but the disease prevalence was relatively higher. It appeared that prevention was not widespread in most systems. Only the Sydney sample gave evidence of successful preventive services and responsive population behavior.

If we look at Figure 20–1, the three study sites in which there are school-based dental care systems (namely, Canterbury, Trøndelag, and·Aarhus), the Aarhus student sample has the lowest DMF score (8.1). Moller reported to the FDI meeting in Athens that the comparable figure ten years ago was 11; he suggested that strong preventive elements in the Aarhus system—fortnightly fluoride mouth rinsing, tooth brushing instruction, motivation efforts, and special attention to high risk groups—probably contributed to this disease reduction. In Canterbury and Trøndelag, the system seems to have been successful from a restorative point of view, but the effect of any preventive effort is difficult to detect.

In the remaining four study sites, which have no systematic school-based delivery system, Baltimore and Sydney are seen to have lower DMF figures than those found in areas covered by systematic school programs. Baltimore has an extremely low DMF score (2.9), perhaps because the water supply has been fluoridated since 1952 and perhaps because blacks, who tend to have lower caries rates than non-blacks, form a relatively large proportion of the sampled population. Sydney's relatively low DMF of 6.7 may result from increases in utilization of dental services in the past decade and perhaps from increased preventive measures in use by dentists, community institutions, and consumers themselves. In systems where recall to the dental office or clinic is not built in, utilization of services seems to be a significant predictor of need for treatment. If a system has regular utilization built into the operation of the program, consumer preventive behavior and perceptions of oral treatment needs become more important predictors of actual treatment needs.

ADULTS

The results of the adult data, reported initially in 1976 at the FDI meetings in Athens, suggest that even the best school dental care system may not be able to effect a satisfactory level of oral health on a long-term basis (see Figure 20-2). It should be remembered, however, that several caries prevention measures applied today were not available at the time these thirty-five to forty-four year olds were in their teens. Even with this caveat, it is interesting to observe that the decay component of the DMF index is 2 or lower in all areas. On the other hand, the missing component is rather high in all areas with the exceptions of Hannover and Yamanashi. The filled component is higher in Aarhus than in any other site, and the total DMF is also higher in Aarhus.

The periodontal index (PI), used in the adult samples (see Table 20-1), revealed a considerable difference between the Hannover, Yamanashi, and Baltimore samples and the other three. Females have consistently lower scores than males. Only the Yamanashi sample, and to a lesser extent the Trøndelag sample, demonstrated a higher PI score for nonmetropolitan data than for metropolitan. None of the means suggests a very high level of periodontal disease, although the possible effect of missing teeth on the periodontal index, at least

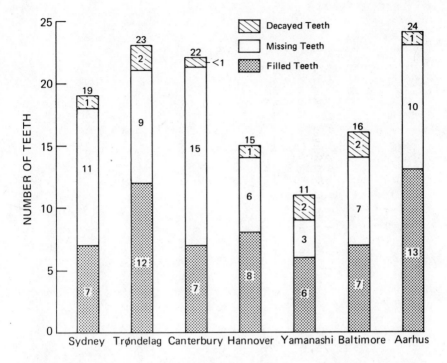

Figure 20–2. DMF Adult Sample of Thirty-five to Forty-four Year Olds, ICSDM Survey. *(In contrast to children of Aarhus, adult DMF component is highest of seven sites. Also note overall low decay but generally high missing components.)*

Source: World Health Organization—Division of Dentistry, International Collaborative Study of Dental Manpower.

for Canterbury and Sydney, should be investigated further. (There was almost no periodontitis—measured by the number of teeth with gingivitis—among the student samples.)

Looking at edentulousness, the terminal stage of caries and periodontal diseases, we see that the percentages of people without any teeth range from 0 in Yamanashi and 2 in Hannover to an extraordinary 36 in Canterbury. Sydney, Baltimore, Aarhus, and Trøndelag are in the middle range (see Table 20–2).

The percentage of the sample who were denture wearers in the Danish study was 31, compared to 14 in Yamanashi, 23 in Hannover, 27 in Trøndelag, 47 and 55 in Sydney and Canterbury, respectively. Thirty-six percent of the Baltimore sample had full or partial dentures. Perhaps the most striking feature in the prosthetic area is that

Table 20–1. Periodontal Index (modified) as Indicator of Adult Oral Health Status from ICSDM Survey. (Worldwide, females have better PI than males. German, Japanese, and American PI index are considerably higher than Australian, Norwegian, and New Zealand.)

	Sydney	Trøndelag	Canterbury	Hannover	Yamanashi	Baltimore
Male	1.37	1.07	1.05	1.80	1.88	1.96
Female	1.10	0.94	0.89	1.66	1.62	1.65
Metropolitan	1.19	0.96	0.99	1.73	1.60	1.97
Non-metropolitan	1.26	1.05	0.95	1.72	1.86	1.59
Both Areas	1.22	1.00	0.97	1.73	1.74	1.78

Source: World Health Organization—Division of Dentistry, International Collaborative Study of Dental Manpower.

Table 20–2. Percent of Edentulous Persons from ICSDM Survey. *(Marked contrast between Canterbury, New Zealand, and Yamanashi, Japan, bears continuing investigation.)*

Sydney	Trønde-lag	Canter-bury	Hannover	Yamanashi	Balti-more	Aarhus
13	6	36	2	0	11	10

Source: World Health Organization— Division of Dentistry, International Collaborative Study of Dental Manpower.

approximately 85 percent of the denture wearers sampled in the Danish study need further prosthetic care as compared with 70 percent in Trøndelag, 68 percent in Baltimore, 60 percent in Canterbury and Sydney, 50 percent in Yamansashi, and 35 percent in Hannover.

RATIOS OF TREATMENT TO NEED

Figure 20–3 is a depiction of one of the outcome (dependent) variables used in the study. The amount of restorative care provided was computed as the ratio of teeth treated to teeth needing treatment. When the teeth treated in the past but requiring retreatment are subtracted, a new ratio is formed—the successful treatment to need ratio. In the student data, these ratios indicate a sharp difference between the two samples in Trøndelag and Canterbury and the other three original samples. The two areas with highly structured school dental services had a high level of successful treatment and relatively low levels of retreatment needed.

Adult unmet needs are greater than student unmet needs in the two systems where there is a school-based service for children. Unmet needs in adults are relatively less than the unmet need for students in all other systems, except in Baltimore, where the two are about equal equal. Nonetheless, the percentage of unmet adult need is least in Canterbury and Trøndelag, greatest in Yamanashi and Baltimore, and intermediate in Sydney and Hannover.

RELATIONSHIP OF CLINICAL
TO SOCIOLOGICAL VARIABLES

Stepwise regression analysis was applied to determine how much clinical variance could be explained by each of the major sociological variables. The effects of utilization were removed before analyzing the student data in order to ensure that the full extent of any direct relationship between the use of services and oral health status would

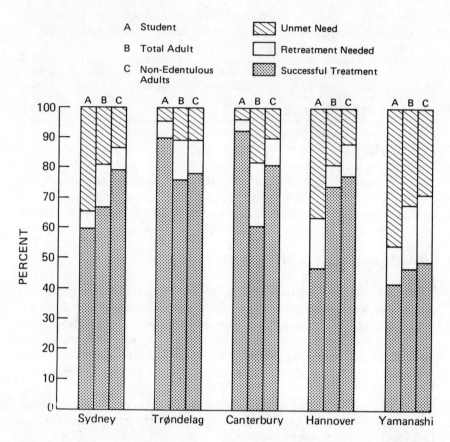

Figure 20–3. Retreatment Needs and Unmet Needs Compared to Successful Treatment in Total Population of ICSDM Survey. *(In student category, Norway and New Zealand ratios far exceed Australia, Germany, and Japan, reflecting strong school-based dental care.)*

Source: World Health Organization—Division of Dentistry, International Collaborative Study of Dental Manpower.

be demonstrated. The sociological variables examined were perception of need, visit behavior, and finally, sociodemographic factors. The same process was used on the adult data, although oral health practice variables were allowed to enter the analysis in competition with perception of need and visit behavior items.

For all seven sets of dependent variables used in this preliminary analysis, there was a remarkable consistency. Just two variables—user type and perceived need for treatment—account for most, and in some cases all, of the variance explained. User type is a measure of utilization frequency and consistency. The perceived need variable results from a yes or no response to the question, If you went to the dentist tomorrow, do you think he would find anything wrong with your teeth or gums? The latter variable is positively associated with the number of missing teeth and the amount of disease present, while the former variable (user type) is negatively associated with these disease measures. Both variables, interestingly enough, represent characteristics of the consumer rather than of the system of organization itself. At this point, I do not know why these two variables are so important. Perhaps future analyses will shed light on the question.

But this finding itself raises other questions. Perhaps availability and accessibility of care do not necessarily ensure utilization of the system or, more to the point, lower levels of unmet need. Whether people can be motivated to visit dental professionals often and consistently, and whether people can be made aware that preventive behavior can preempt the need for prosthetic care appear to be major, not minor, concerns for the professional dental community and for public administrators. While policymakers debate such issues as auxiliary utilization, overspecialization, and manpower training, perhaps the real issue is that oral health status seems to be more closely affected by consumer behavior and beliefs than by manpower arrangements.

SOME POLICY ISSUES

It is too early in the analysis to make public policy recommendations, but the preliminary data do raise some issues:

The Value of Dual Systems
for Children and Adults

While the student data from the two highly structured, school-based dental care systems reveal that this kind of organizational approach can result in very low levels of unmet need for students, the amount of unmet need from adult samples in those same areas approximates that found in two other systems where children do not receive special treatment. Why is this so? Are double systems, with differential services for children and adults, appropriate?

Perhaps any special dental services that are provided should be made available for all age groups, with reinforcing messages given to parents and children alike in the same environment and under similar conditions. It may be easier for a public official to organize an incremental program for school children, adding one academic grade a year until all grades are covered, but does that incremental plan place the child, siblings, and parents at a disadvantage because each is exposed to different messages and different stimuli, and some are exposed to no dental health incentives at all? The discrepancy between the pragmatism of organizing easy to reach school populations and the idea that oral health outcome may be the product of extradental influences, such as the family, ought to concern us when we array the data for further hypothesis testing.

Factors Predicting Utilization

If there is a direct relationship between utilization of dental services and oral health—that is, the more one visits for dental services, the less the unmet need or the better one's oral health—then we need to ask which factors predict utilization. Is income a factor? One would not think so, since previous studies have shown that education (though it is correlated with income) seems to be more strongly related to at least the preventive aspects of utilization; the Danish replication appears to provide further evidence of this association. Travel time, especially in rural areas, has not been important if the need perceived by people impels them to attend care facilities. Perceived need is also strongly associated with care utilization. Further analyses—which will feed in measures of availability of care, access to care, and acceptability—may diminish, enhance, or leave unchanged the importance of perceived need.

If perceived need continues to be the most important predictor, and if we can prove that high utilization services result in better treatment to need ratios, then the policy implication is that planners must contemplate large-scale educational programs to persuade the public of its individual unmet oral health needs and that they must present those needs to dental care professionals. The public's motivation to seek care appears to be an essential component, particularly in the open systems where dental visits are not required and if optimal oral health is the issue. While the dental profession acknowledges the importance of such consumer-oriented efforts, the paucity of resources allocated and expended worldwide on research, development, and demonstration of effective consumer educational activities is testimony either to lip service or to real doubts about the significance of the consumer's role in maintaining his own oral health.

When the data on reasons people visited dental professionals were examined, not all systems demonstrated similar patterns. There appear to be some incentives for preventive utilization in the Trøndelag situation that would be worth exploring further. Fifty-four percent of the Trøndelag adult sample visited the dentist for preventive reasons. All the other samples, as well as public opinion data for U.S. adults over the past few years, demonstrate that only about one-third of the respondents visit for preventive reasons. And in Yamanashi, fully 89 percent of the sample visited for symptomatic reasons.

The Mystery of Edentulousness

Further evidence that these data illustrate the importance of consumer behavior is provided by the finding that tooth loss does not bear a close relationship to disease prevalence patterns. Something seems to be happening in the interaction between the consumer and provider of dental services that results in more tooth loss than might be expected on the basis of observed disease prevalence. Are consumers demanding extractions? Are providers extracting more teeth than they should? What incentives for extraction exist in a particular system?

Results from the first five countries on satisfaction with the condition of one's mouth show close correlation with the percentages of edentulousness in each sample area. The more edentulous a population, the more satisfied they appear to be. While it is startling to learn that people may actually like edentulousness, the dental profession can hardly accept that level of care. We are again alerted that consumer-related information may be an important determinant of how successful the dental profession can be. All too often, policymakers concentrate on different ways to arrange dental providers, where to house them, and what to charge the patient or insuring body. But the consumer has more to say about whether he ever physically appears for care than most planners are willing to recognize. The implication, then, is to place more emphasis on consumer issues than on provider issues when discussing the organizational aspects of dental care delivery.

Quality of Care

The need for retreatment apparently differs widely among the samples. Certainly, these data need further examination to shed light on questions of quality of care and on why retreatment needs are high or low from place to place. Do some dental delivery systems regard quantity rather than quality to varying degrees?

PROSPECTS

It should be emphasized that we have not aimed for exact comparability, free of measurement error, because the sciences involved are not yet sophisticated enough to deal with variations of disease and health definitions, let alone other related variables, across cultures. We have been concerned with those aspects of systems that can be changed—not those aspects that, for one reason or another, are unchangeable. Furthermore, we could not possibly study all potentially relevant information across cultures. Sheer limits of human power prevent computerization of all the elements that may be related to oral health outcomes.

But, with all these limitations—and many more associated with language learning, disciplinary jargons, locating common research talent across systems, maintaining contented staff for extended periods, insufficient funds to commit staff full-time for long duration—the binding agents for the collaboration, nonetheless, have remained secure. Those bonds of collaboration—national interest, government commitment, commonality of practical objectives, involvement of a neutral international organization that can facilitate communication across sociopolitical interests, recognition of the equality of skill contribution across disciplines, and, perhaps most important of all, tremendous human will and physical effort—provide us with a recipe for collaboration that sustains this continuing effort and that, one may hope, will stimulate other international dental research projects.

ABOUT THE AUTHOR

Dr. Lois Cohen is special assistant to the director of the National Institute of Dental Research at the National Institutes of Health. Before joining the NIDR, she was special assistant to the director of the USPHS Division of Dentistry and served as chief of the Office of Social and Behavioral Analysis with the division. More important to this report, Dr. Cohen was one of the directors of the international study on which she so ably reports.

Dr. Cohen received her B.A. degree in sociology from the University of Pennsylvania and both her Master's and Ph.D. degrees in sociology from Purdue.

Her present address is: 9000 Rockville Pike, Building #31, Room 2C-39, Bethesda, Maryland 20014.

Chapter 21

The Effect of Plaque Control in Sweden— A Preventive Experience

Dr. Jan Erik Ahlberg

I have been asked by my U.S. colleague, Dr. John Ingle, to report on some recent research on the effect of a plaque control program on caries, gingivitis, and progressive periodontal disease. This research was carried out by Professor Jan Lindhe and Dr. Per Axelsson in Sweden and is undoubtedly of enormous significance in the world-wide fight against these diseases.

THE TRIAL WITH SCHOOL CHILDREN

The first trial was initiated in 1971, testing the hypothesis that dental caries and gingivitis will not develop in school children maintained on an oral hygiene program that includes meticulous professional tooth cleaning and oral hygiene instruction once every second week. Three age groups of Swedish children, seven to eight, ten to eleven, and thirteen to fourteen, all from the same school in Karlstad, were selected for the study. Initially, a baseline examination was carried out, establishing indexes of dental plaque, gingival inflammation, and dental caries for each child. The 216 children were then evenly and arbitrarily assigned into test and control groups. The thirteen to four-teen year old children had all experienced a high caries attack rate—a "high risk group." Over the four years under investigation, only 5 percent of the children were lost from the study per year.

The preventive program for the control groups included supervised tooth brushing once a month with an 0.2 percent sodium fluoride solution. The test group children, on the other hand, were taught the use of toothbrush and dental floss, following plaque-staining with red dye disclosing tablets. More important for the result, all surfaces of the teeth were cleaned by specially trained dental assistants (pro-phydental nurses). Plaque was removed with an abrasive paste containing 5 percent monofluorophosphate. Both dental floss and brushes were used interproximally, the latter in a special reciprocating handpiece. A regular rotary handpiece mounted with rubber cups or brushes was used on smooth or occlusal surfaces. For two years during the school year, "professional" tooth cleaning was carried out every two weeks (except during the three month summer holiday) requiring about ten to fifteen minutes each time.

Caries

At the end of the first and second years, the test and control groups were reexamined. The results were startling. At one year, all the children together in the test group had developed only six new carious lesions, while the same size control group had developed 300 lesions—fifty times more decay. At the end of two years, the experimentals had only nineteen new cavities. The controls had over 600—thirty times more. Over a three year period, the ninety-three children in the test group developed a total of only 42 new carious surfaces, while the controls developed 790 new lesions—nearly twenty times more. In the four years of the study, the test group developed only 61 new carious lesions, whereas the controls developed 941—over fifteen times as many cavities (Figure 21–1).

Plaque and Gingival Index

The same amazing difference became apparent in the plaque and gingival indexes. A plaque index score of two indicates visible bacterial plaque at the gingival line of the tooth. Initially, over 20 percent of all the children, test and control, had such a plaque index score. After one and two years, however, less than 1 percent of the test group children had a plaque index score of two, whereas the control group children remained essentially the same as at their initial examination—around 20 percent. At the end of the third and fourth years, twice as many test children (70 percent) had all tooth surfaces free form plaque as did the control children (35 percent) (Figure 21–2).

A low plaque index is associated with a low gingival inflammation score. After one and two years of "professional" tooth cleaning, not a single gingival unit among the test group was moderately inflamed (Gingival Inflammation score—two). On the other hand, 10 percent of the gingiva of the control group remained severely inflamed; and

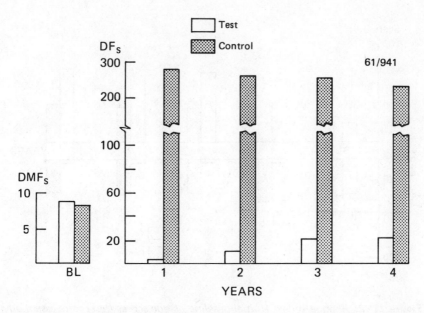

Figure 21–1. Total Number of New Carious Surfaces. *(In baseline study, left, test and control groups started out the same. In four years, test groups had developed only 61 new carious surfaces whereas controls had developed nearly 1,000 new carious surfaces.)*

Source: Dr. Per Axelsson, author, and Dr. Nathaniel H. Rowe, editor, *Proceedings of Symposium on the Scientific Basis for Evaluation of Periodontal Therapy* (Ann Arbor: University of Michigan, 1977), used with permission.

by the end of three years, marked gingival inflammation involved 20 percent of all control group gingival units (Figure 21–3).

During the third year of the study, the intervals between the sessions of "professional" tooth cleaning were extended from two weeks to four weeks for the younger children and to eight weeks for the thirteen to fourteen year old "high risk" adolescents. During the fourth year, the intervals were prolonged to two months in groups one and two and to three to four months for group three—only three to four sessions a year. Even with this dramatic change in professional attention, the test groups maintained 70 percent of all permanent tooth surfaces free of dental plaque, whereas the controls did not improve from their initial examination four years before.

In the fourth and final year, the test group children developed only 0.28 filled or decayed surfaces per child. Only one hour of prophylactic treatment per child per year was expended to achieve this

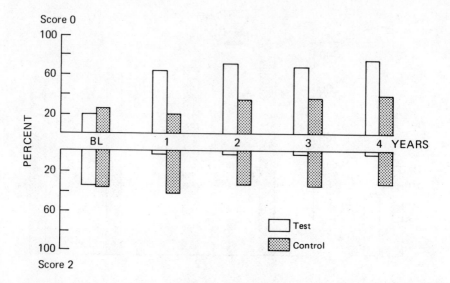

Figure 21−2. Plaque Index. *(Initial baseline plaque scores (left) were essentially the same between test and control groups. In four years, significant differences developed between groups. Virtually none of test group had a plaque score of 2 (below line). In addition, 70 percent developed a plaque index of 0 (above line). Control groups did not improve.)*

Source: Dr. Per Axelsson, author, and Dr. Nathaniel H. Rowe, editor, *Symposium on the Scientific Basis for Evaluation of Periodontal Therapy* (Ann Arbor, University of Michigan, 1977), used with permission.

result—and the cost was only 54 Swedish crowns, or about $13, per child. One full-time prophydental nurse could, in fact, almost completely prevent caries and gingivitis for 1,000 Swedish school children. Translated into twenty years of intact teeth with no perio-dontal disease, such a program (over twenty years) would require seven hours of diagnosis and orthodontic treatment by a dentist and twenty-five hours of preventive treatment by an auxiliary. The twenty year cost for such a program is around 2,600 Swedish crowns, or only $606 per person—$30 a year.

A number of studies of similar design, including crossover trials, where the control and test groups are switched halfway through the study, have confirmed the results.

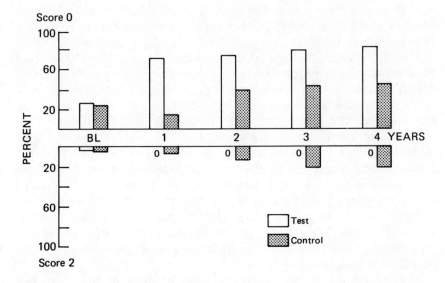

Figure 21—3. Gingival Index. *(Although test and control groups started at same levels (left, "BL"), no gingival inflammation was detected in test groups after one year, whereas control groups showed little improvement.)*

Source: Dr. Per Axelsson, author, and Dr. Nathaniel H. Rowe, editor, *Proceedings of Symposium on the Scientific Basis for Evaluation of Periodontal Therapy* (Ann Arbor, University of Michigan, 1977), used with permission.

THE TRIAL WITH ADULTS

A second trial, an investigation on adults, was carried out to determine if the occurrence of caries and the progression of periodontitis can be prevented in adults who are maintained at a proper oral hygiene standard by regular instruction and prophylaxis. An attempt was also made in the trial to study the progression of dental diseases in individuals who received no special oral hygiene instruction but received regular dental care of a traditional type.

Three different age groups of individuals from one geographic site were recruited in 1971–1972 for the trial; 330 were assigned to a test and 180 to a control group. A baseline examination revealed that the socioeconomic status, the oral hygiene status, the incidence of gingivitis, and the caries experience were similar in both test and control participants prior to the start of the study.

During the subsequent three year period, the control patients were seen regularly once a year and given traditional dental care. The test group participants, on the other hand, were seen once every two months during the first two years and once every three months during the third year. At each appointment, on an individual basis, they were instructed in proper oral hygiene technique and given a careful dental prophylaxis including scaling and root planing. Each prophylactic session was conducted by a dental hygienist. A reexamination was carried out toward the end of the third treatment year.

At the reexamination three years later, the oral hygiene status of all three test groups had markedly improved in comparison with the baseline data. Thus, the total mean plaque score had decreased from 62.4 percent to 17.4 percent (young adults, Group I), 61.9 percent to 19.1 percent (middle age, Group II), and from 63.0 percent to 17.8 percent (older, Group III). This decrease in the plaque scores was statistically significant ($p < 0.001$) for each group. In the control groups, there was no obvious improvement between the initial and final examination.

Concomitant with the improved oral hygiene of the three test groups at the reexamination, the gingival inflammation scores were markedly reduced. The frequency of inflamed gingival units had decreased from 22.2 percent to 1.7 percent (Group I), 20.6 percent to 1.3 percent (Group II), and 24.7 percent to 2.0 percent (Group III). The degree of improvement of the gingival condition was similar in all three groups of patients and highly significant ($p < 0.00$). In fact, the gingival-bleeding scores of only 1 to 2 percent indicated that the test group patients had clinically healthy gingivae. In the control groups, on the other hand, there was no obvious improvement in the number of gingival units that bled following gentle probing during the observation period.

In the test groups, there was a significant reduction of clinical pocket depth between the baseline examination and reexamination. The mean pocket depths decreased from 2.0 to 1.5 mm (Group I), 3.1 to 1.4 mm (Group II), and from 3.2 to 1.5 mm (Group III). More important, in all age groups, the pocket depth reduction was most pronounced in the interdental areas. In the control groups, there was a corresponding slight increase of pocket depth (Group I, 0.5 mm; Group II, 0.6 mm; Group III, 0.5 mm) between the two examinations.

As one might suspect from the pocket depth studies, there was a corresponding difference in the clinical attachment levels between the baseline examination and the reexamination three years later (Figure 21–4). In the test groups, there were no alterations of the

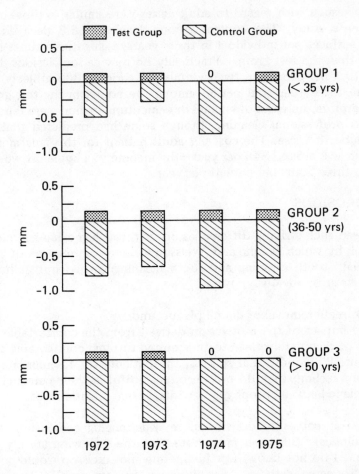

Figure 21—4. Attachment Level Alterations in Adults, 1972—1975. *(Whereas test groups show improvement in attachment levels, control groups show considerable loss.)*

attachment level. In all three control groups, however, the clinical attachment level had shifted apically. In control Group I, the loss of attachment amounted to 0.5 mm. The corresponding figures for control Groups II and III were 0.8 and 0.9, respectively. This means that, whereas the test group patients were able to maintain the level of their periodontal tissues, the control patients, over the three year period, lost significant amounts of their attachment apparatus. There was a tendency among the older control patients (fifty to sixty-five years old) to lose attachment at a faster rate than younger individuals.

The results with regard to adult caries were similar to those in the children's study. The control groups developed 8.3 decayed and filled surfaces per individual in three years, eighty-three times more caries than the test groups. Practically no new carious lesions developed (0.1 per person, or twenty-nine new caries in 330 subjects) during the three year trial period among the adults in the test group. Furthermore, no cases of enamel or cementum erosion were reported due to professional cleaning, though some had predicted that this would be the case. The cost per adult patient for this treatment in Sweden was around $40 per year—the income of a hygienist working two to three hours per patient per year.

CONCLUSIONS

How can such striking differences occur through mechanical plaque control, by which Lindhe and Axelsson mean a combination of "professional" tooth cleaning and tooth cleaning carried out at home? The answer is, obviously, by:

1. Complete removal of dental plaque; and
2. The impact of the motivation derived from the comfortable feeling of completely clean teeth acquired through comfortable treatment. With individual success, the patients try to maintain this clean feeling; they do not become slothful in their personal oral hygiene between prophylactic visits, as one might expect.

When it comes to drawing more wide-ranging conclusions from these clinical trials, you must note that the following are my own and that I do not know how far Lindhe and Axelsson would be prepared to agree with me. Swedish scientists are usually, and quite rightly, cautious about drawing conclusions that are not entirely supported by firm scientific evidence. In my position, on the other hand, I feel justified in making even provocative statements in order to bring about discussion and some fresh thinking.

On the basis of the assembled mass of experiences from the delivery system and clinical field trials in Sweden, I would state the following:

1. The investigations of Lindhe and Axelsson demonstrate that every person responsible for planning oral health care delivery must, first of all, include disease prevention by means of plaque control as the very basic concept of any delivery system.

2. Efficient plaque control can be managed with the aid of auxiliaries, who need only limited training. In the Lindhe and Axelsson study, the chairside assistants needed only five or six weeks of special training. In the words of Axelsson, however, they must be "well motivated, responsible, and skillful."[1]

Some conclusions have relevance primarily for the industrialized countries. Among these are that:

1. Reparative-prosthetic treatment is time consuming, demanding in manpower, and therefore expensive. It also produces only a limited reduction, if any, in the volume of oral diseases.

2. Plans to introduce dental health insurance schemes based primarily on subsidizing reparative treatment or to introduce new categories of operating auxiliaries with mainly reparative functions are based on priorities that may have seemed relevant ten to fifteen years ago but are of doubtful value today.

3. The most useful categories of auxiliaries to bring about plaque control, and thereby disease prevention, are the two most commonly found in the industrialized countries—namely, the dental (chairside) assistant and the dental hygienist. The application of mechanical plaque control in the dental office does not require sophisticated facilities, and its complete success is closely related to the motivation of the individual. Plaque control would, therefore, seem to be easily adaptable to many different systems of delivery without great interference in their present general structure.

In developing countries, where a real delivery system may hardly exist, an adequate solution might involve a mixture of different approaches. One hundred years ago, Sweden was almost a developing country as far as dentistry was concerned. Since then, dentistry has passed through three main stages of development: (1) relief of pain, (2) replacement of lost teeth, and (3) a reparative stage; it has recently entered into the fourth, or preventive, stage. The scarcity of resources and the rapid increase in oral diseases may emphasize that present-day developing countries, while of necessity alloting resources to stages one and two, should preferably try to bypass stage three and jump directly to stage four.

Finally, I would like to emphasize one further important factor, which dentists have long understood worldwide, but which they may not adequately have conveyed to planners and politicians—in particular, to those who wish to develop the right priorities in spending public money for dental services. This quotation from an excellent Swedish continuing education course for the dental team on oral disease prevention, points in the right direction. It is a conversation between a dentist and a patient: "There are 8,760 hours in a year. You spend perhaps two hours in the dentist's chair. This means that it is up to you to care for your teeth for the other 8,758 hours of the year. Agreed?"

NOTES

1. Per Axelsson, Evaluation of periodontal therapy: Longitudinal clinical trials in Sweden, in *Proceedings of Symposium on The Scientific Basis for Evaluation of Periodontal Therapy*, (Ann Arbor: University of Michigan School of Dentistry, October 1976), pp. 36–39.

ABOUT THE AUTHOR

Dr. Ahlberg is presently the executive director of the Federation Dentaire Internationale, with headquarters in London. Prior to his rather recent acceptance of this international assignment, he was executive director of the Swedish Dental Federation. As such he had a good deal to do with helping direct Sweden's efforts in the delivery of dental care as well as with formulating policy for the future.

Dr. Ahlberg received his dental degree (Leg. Tandlakare) from the Faculty of Odontology at the Karolinska Institute in Stockholm.

His present address is: 64 Wimpole Street, London W1m 8AL, England.

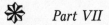 *Part VII*

Audience Participation

Two question and answer sessions were recorded. Over two hours of transcribed material was edited for clarity and brevity to form this chapter. The editors have made every effort to in no way change the meaning of either the questions or the answers.

Chapter 22

Edited Question
and Answer Sessions

Q. *DR. ALVIN MORRIS*, Association for Academic Health Centers: Dr. Logan, I'd be interested to know the tenure of employment of the New Zealand dental nurses. Also, how many drop out to attend dental school?

A. *DR. LOGAN*: Our information here is quite clear, with big changes appearing at the moment. For many years, we averaged a career life for dental nurses of about six or seven years. About 1974, a change started, and now the average work span of a New Zealand dental nurse has increased to about ten years. It's still going up, and we don't know where it will stop. But a part of the change is that the ability to control family size, the wish to have smaller families, and the wish of women to remain longer in the work force have reached new levels. Career life for a dental nurse may continue climbing to fifteen, sixteen, maybe even twenty years.

As far as the number entering dentistry, so far we've only had one graduate from dentistry. We've encouraged a number, but they seem to find their present career reasonably satisfying. In the last analysis of the dental registry, 1.7 percent of the registered dentists were women, but a very big change has occurred since 1975, and now about 30 percent of the recruits to dentistry are women.

Q. *DR. MILTON LINSANSKY*, Yale University: Dr. Logan, you stated that forceps have been removed from the school dental nurse armamentarium. Do you think that if forceps were removed from the New Zealand dentists, it might have any effect on the outcome of the program?

A. *DR. LOGAN*:   No comment (audience laughter).

Q. *DR. HARVEY WEBB*, president of the National Dental Association: In America we have approximately forty million under-served and poor people who fall into a category similar to those identified in many other countries. Today I've heard several success stories that seem to indicate that something can be done that's effective and compatible with the population. I would like Drs. Cohen and Schoen to answer this question: To what degree are the things being done in other countries applicable in America as it relates to human reactions and the state of dental practice and sophistication here?

A. *DR. COHEN*:   That's a very large question. First of all, in order to suggest options that might be successful for this population, we must first seek to identify the characteristics of the forty million people of whom you speak. Many of the examples of innovative ideas we have heard today deal with rural populations. But I don't know that the forty million underserved in the United States are all in rural areas. We have pockets in urban concentrations that are equally underserved. The idea of transplanting one model from one culture to another doesn't make sense to me, except on an experimental basis, to see whether successful features from the other models, combined in our own cultural context, make any sense. We must then evaluate outcomes.

I was fascinated to see and hear about the Mexican idea of taking the service to the people, as a home-to-home service. There have been services in mobile units taken to communities, but the idea of taking a service to the family seems to be a unique idea. This would fit with certain notions of consumer behavior—that is, people do those things to which they have been exposed throughout their life and family experience. We must begin to think about the idea of the family as the unit of care rather than the individual. The Mexican chapter (see Chapter 8) suggested a sociological concept that may have relevance to dentistry.

A. *DR. SCHOEN*: Please remember, Dr. Webb, that we also have some background in this country for programs that have worked —successful demonstration type programs that have been phased out or that covered only relatively small populations but then were never extended to others. I'd like to add one point to Dr. Cohen's remarks. One of the thoughts I've had, particularly after listening today, is to try taking a school-based situation and extend it to the whole family. Schools generally are located convenient to population and with some kind of a relationship to population. If school-based programs can be extended back to the whole family, then maybe we'll bridge some of the gap which now seems to occur after the children leave school. There are obviously some troubles with this, however, because not all of the children in one family go to the same school.

We really don't need to look very far to know that we should have someone like a dental nurse. Maybe we should stop training hygienists and start training dental nurses instead, and then have them perform functions not just on school children, but on adults as well. Certainly, they could be taught to perform the intraoral and direct personal service functions of making dentures. This would require fewer dentists. It would be easy for us, with our resources, to switch over to other types of providers.

One last point. The way dentists are trained, I don't think we dentists can really do a proper job with prevention. We get our kicks from doing complicated things, and not from prevention. We're disease-oriented, not health-oriented, and I'm speaking about myself now. I think that developing behavior change in patients has to be dealt with by other personnel, again in organized situations. Some of this comes through from what we've heard today. In our country, I consider it a shame that we have to think and talk about this at this time. With the kinds of resources we have, we should be beyond it.

Q. *DR. NEIL DEMBY*, Lutheran Medical Center, New York City: Dr. Schoen, some observers believe that a health system really mirrors the political and economic system in any country. In light of this observation, how do you perceive that any definitive changes might be made in our dental system without equal changes [being made] in the political and economic system of this country?

A. *DR. SCHOEN*: True, the way you practice dentistry or health
care in general is related to the politics and the economy of the
country. However, we do know that there are countries with political and economic systems not terribly different from ours that
have different health care systems. Although I don't think a major political change is going to occur here tomorrow, I do think it
is possible, within the health care system, to make some major
changes. I'm not prepared to give up on radical change in one
system while waiting for a change in the other, which will happen
long after I'm dead and gone.

Q. *DR. ALVIN MORRIS*: Dr. Miyares, in Cuba you have experienced a change in a political system and in the health system. Do
you think it is possible to modify the health system without a
corresponding modification of the political system? Does the experience in Cuba support that?

A. *DR. MIYARES*: My impression is that, without political change,
it is very difficult to introduce real changes in the welfare system.

A. *DR. GILLESPIE*: It has just occurred to me that in this region
of the Americas there are thirty-one countries. We have just been
presented with the example of changes in the health systems of
Cuba and Ecuador. Both countries are going the same way, dentally speaking, but they're completely opposed politically. Some
health components come through irrespective of the political system. It's really a question of national administration rather than
political approach.

Q. *DR. ERNEST HARDAWAY*, U.S. Public Health Service: Dr.
Schoen, you mentioned the fabrication of dentures, and someone
from the audience mentioned lack of access for the nonprivileged
communities. I'd like to pose this question. What impact do you
feel a broad or universal financing mechanism might have on
access for nonprivileged people, both regarding dentures and
bringing health services into the nonprivileged community?

A. *DR. SCHOEN*: I think it would depend upon the system. If
only the method of payment is changed, and not the administrative and organizational arrangements, it might have a very limited
impact or the kind of spotty, up and down, good and bad impact
of Medicaid and Medicare. With appropriate administration, appropriate financing, appropriate incentives for delivery changes, a

universal financing mechanism could have a major impact upon health delivery as well as [on] the consequent oral health of the population.

A. *DR. GILLESPIE*:   In regard to the specific reference to dentures and the underprivileged, we must go back to problems emanating from dental education. I would imagine that in 90 percent of the dental schools in the world, when a denture is made for some-body, the patient will have to make five or six visits. It's very apparent to me that this is a pretty unacceptable system for many people who have to take time out from employment, who have problems of transportation to the dentist's office, and who then might have to wait in the office to be seen. This is simply not an acceptable approach.

   In some of our denture programs, particularly in rural areas, we have started to design it differently—taking a hint from what the empiricists (quacks) were doing, and then we patterning the sys-tem differently. Basically, the change was to complete two or three stages at one time and then to have the person return at the second appointment for the finished product. It has been gratify-ing to see the community acceptance of this kind of approach.

Q. *DR. SHELDON ROVIN*, University of Washington. This ques-tion is directed to Dr. Baz, from Mexico, and Dr. Miyares, from Cuba. I believe we can accept the concept that what happens in health care in a given country is a reflection of its social values. It's my impression that many people in the United States are apathetic toward health care, particularly dental care. Some of the success stories you portrayed to us seem to reflect a different attitude of people from Mexico and Cuba. Specifically, what are the general and social attitudes in Latin America regarding dental care?

A. *DR. MIYARES*:   I will talk about our experience in Cuba. Sev-enteen years ago, before the revolution, about 30 percent of the Cuban people were illiterate. Now there is no illiteracy. The cul-ture has gone up, and people now expect a high level in medical and dental care. There is a demand by all the population. Years ago they asked only for extractions. Now, they don't like ex-tractions. They ask now for fillings, for prosthetic dentistry, and for orthodontic treatment for their children. I suspect that when a country has more development, people ask for more sophisti-cated things.

A. *DR. BAZ*: I agree with Dr. Miyares. I think it's a question of education. One finds in scattered populations that when they have a toothache, they don't try to cure it, because they have to pay for what they need to have done. As soon as one starts to work with and educate the community, a demand for services starts and continues to grow. That's how people react. It's education, not political problems, not economic problems.

Q. *DR. JOHN HEIN*, Forsyth Clinic, Boston: Dr. Logan, I've recently been informed that there was a revolt of the New Zealand nurses, that they were making a move to take over the operation without the influence and supervision of dentists. Has that been exaggerated? Could you tell us what is actually going on, because I'm sure that could be a big concern to all sides in this country. The other question I'd like to ask you is, it's perfectly obvious that, in spite of a heavy emphasis on oral health education since 1921, your program has been a total failure in terms of getting the dentists and adult population interested in continuing with a high level of oral health. Have you done anything to modify oral health education or are you going to throw it out and just concentrate on treatment? Have you any new ideas to make it more effective?

A. *DR. LOGAN*: To answer your second question first, I couldn't agree that dental health education has been a total waste; nor could I claim that our health education has been successful. At the same time, I'm not aware of any country in the world that has achieved much success in the field of health education. As far as the different components of our program are concerned, we first went through an era when we were relieving pain. We then went through an era when we were removing carious tissue and restoring teeth, and now we're into an era where the emphasis is going toward prevention. We expect to see a very considerable drop in the very near future in the need for restorative care. We have set ourselves an objective for 1977 to reduce the need for restorations by 10 percent, and it looks as if we will achieve it. We are also diversifying the program to meet the needs of local communities. It was a standardized program, but we're now diversifying according to local disease patterns.

   In answer to your first question, as far as the so-called revolt is concerned, I know of no great revolt. In 1974–1975, we faced a situation where our school dental nurses were being manipulated by their union—the public service association. This union was upset by a white paper that had been published on a future health organization for New Zealand. They feared that all the health people, 47,000—50,000 members, would move out of the union and form an organization of their own. So the union set out to manipulate one or two groups. The dental nurse group was pretty naive, and they got manipulated. To them, it appeared to be a salary issue, for which procedure is well established. They didn't go through the procedure, but it was resolved quite happily in the end.

Q. *DR. ROBIN LAWRENCE*, U.S. Public Health Service, Boston: I'm interested in the cost of comprehensive care for children. I would like to get from the panel the per child cost in each of your programs. Dr. Lewis, of Canada, indicated a cost of about $107 per child, and I guess, if you take out the depreciation for capital equipment, the cost per child would be about $102. Can we have similar cost figures for other countries, in whatever currency is appropriate?

A. *DR. BAZ*: Well, the treatment our technicians give in Mexico will cost us under $7—the whole treatment per child.

A. *DR. LOGAN*: First of all, we have to put this in some sort of perspective. I heard this morning that the average net income of a U.S. dentist is about $36,000. In New Zealand, the average net income for a dentist is about $19,000—20,000. The salary for an experienced school dental nurse after five years is about $8,000. Well, with that background, the cost of providing care for children from ages two and a half to thirteen is $16.92 (U.S.) per year per child, and the cost under the Dental Benefits Program, providing for children ages thirteen to eighteen, is $25.40 (U.S.) per year.

A. *DR. MIYARES*: I have no complete answer for that question. However, I can speak about the preventive phase of our dental program. Prevention in Cuba costs about 28 cents yearly per child.

A. *DR. LEWIS*: In the second year of the Saskatchewan program, I quoted a total cost of $107 per child, reduced by depreciation of $4.36 down to about $102. On the other hand, if we take the services we provided during the second year of the plan, and cost them out at the Saskatchewan College of Dental Surgeons fee schedule, and then deduct 10 percent (because, when we hire a private practice dentist, we deduct 10 percent of their fee schedule), the value of the services comes out to $116 per child. I think that kind of puts it in some perspective.

Q. *DR. SAUL KAMEN*, Long Island Jewish-Hillside Medical Center: It has been said that the two biggest detriments to dental care in our country are fear and money. It seems to me that some countries are eliminating the financial deterrent to dental care. From this I have two basic questions. First, in your countries has there also been a change in the cultural view of the dentist as a person to be feared? Second, what is the economic level of the dental profession in your countries where you have developed social systems of dental care?

A. *DR. LOGAN*: Of course, it's always said that the two barriers are cost in terms of finance and pain. I think there are many other barriers, also. Some were just mentioned a moment ago: the time spent in the dentist's presence, the inconvenience, the discomfort, the travel costs, the time spent in travel. There are many other barriers. I don't think pain is a big factor in my country. As far as income is concerned, as I stated before, New Zealand dentists average about $20,000 a year.

A. *DR. MIYARES*: As far as people being afraid to go to the dentist, I suppose it's a matter of education. I have seen in our program, from nursery school to primary school, that only a small number of children are afraid of dentists. In the future, they will be very good oral program patients. In regard to the fee, in our country it is free. It is only necessary to pay a small amount for prosthetic dentistry.

A. *DR. BAZ*: With this approach of using dental technicians with children, we have seen that they don't fear to come to us. They are happy to visit the modules, and they let the technicians treat them with no tears and no fears.

A. *DR. LEWIS*: Perhaps just about the fear aspect. You have to understand that it gets cold in Saskatchewan, and there are quite a few days during the school year when the children can't go out at their recess and play on the playground. As I noted in Chapter 7, I found that, more and more, as I visited clinics, if it was a bad day, children were coming down to the dental clinics during the recess and watching the dental nurse restore teeth. There was obviously no fear. More importantly, they were really understanding something about the importance of dental health and how dental disease could be prevented. I think these are perhaps the most important lessons we can teach children, so I'm happy to have them gather in the dental clinic.

Q. *DR. ALLEN HINDIN*, Danbury, Connecticut: I gather that the use of the auxiliary was an asset in helping break down the concept of fear and that the idea of treating the child in a school setting, rather than in a satellite operation, breaks down fear. Fear is very important, but I think cost is of much more concern to people. In my state, a three month to two year backlog currently exists at public health facilities, except for emergency care. A list that size, I think, indicates a great desire and a lack of fear.

What I was wondering was whether any of the gentlemen from outside the United States experienced problems in terms of resistant attitudes from professional associations in terms of licensing? Do you have state by state licensing, as we do? Is there a national license? If you had difficulties, how did you overcome them? Was the dental profession supportive or did they have no choice?

A. *DR. BAZ*: They had no choice. As I explained in Chapter 8, there is a group of people who can pay who go to the dentist. We are working for the people who cannot pay. Originally, the dentists attacked the project, but now they don't mind, because we work on those who can't pay. But even with that, the dentists had no choice but to accept the program.

A. *DR. GILLESPIE*: Of course, there have been a lot of battles and attempts to sabotage programs in certain places. However, what one realizes is that, first of all, some governments in Latin America have much more of a social conscience. They may not always be able to deliver, but at least they express a commitment to provide help for people. Consequently, the organized dental profession is really a very minor force compared with the major governmental political force. At the point of confrontation, the dental association realizes it's fighting a losing battle. You also have to remember that, in developing countries, it's the local practitioner—I won't call him a quack, I'll call him an empiricist or a local practitioner—who has a community base. And because he has a community base, he also has a political base. Often the person with the weakest political base in the community is the professional.

Some of the countries have laws that sound very similar to laws here, laws saying that nobody other than the qualified dentist, with a registered degree from a recognized university, can practice dentistry. But the last half of the sentence often says, "where there is no dentist, anybody can practice." And in some of these countries, the quacks outnumber the professionals three or four to one. And so, the real challenge is how to honor the commitment of the government to provide health care and at the same time produce a quality service under an organized system.

I know that the state dental practice acts in the U.S. are very strict on students working on patients outside university facilities. But I am convinced that there are ways that those practice acts could be suitably modified or amended to allow dental students to have more community experience, and I don't mean just isolated extramural visits of one or two days, but the actual living experience. We're always concerned that the learning dentist or auxiliary is going to do something terrible to the patient. But, in actual fact, in over five years of experience in these programs in Venezuela, I have realized that a dental graduate with community experience is much more capable of producing dental care for the population than one who graduates from a traditional school.

Q. *DR. MORRIS*:   Dr. Logan, has the role of the New Zealand Dental Society in relation to your program been a smooth one?

A. *DR. LOGAN*:   Back in 1921, the origin of our program was the dental profession. Granted, it was some of their strong leaders, but they were the executive officers in the New Zealand Dental Association. So, now we're able to say, "Look, it's your program, your idea."

Q. *ANONYMOUS*:   Dr. Ahlberg, in the Lindhe-Axelsson studies, professional prophylaxis was done. I wonder whether you would expect the same results if the prophylaxis was done by the patients themselves? My second question, would you tell us how you arrived at the 1 to 500 ratio for dentists to population in Sweden?

A. *DR. AHLBERG*:   With regard to professional tooth cleaning as opposed to self-applied tooth cleaning, the two types of tooth cleaning must support each other. It is the experience from these and other investigations that it is in fact very difficult for a patient to achieve 100 percent effective self-applied tooth cleaning without prior help from the professionals. Once they have received a completely plaque-free mouth, however, they are likely to keep it that way for a considerable time. That's why it was possible to extend the periods between the professional tooth cleaning without gross deterioration of the results in the study. From a cost-effectiveness aspect, this must be investigated further.

With regard to the number of dentists in Sweden, I have been personally convinced for quite a long time that the number planned for, up to the end of this century, will prove to be excessive. All the more so if we succeed in using dental assistants to an increasing extent to perform professional tooth cleaning. At present, however, the situation is disguised by the rapid increase in demand caused by the dental insurance scheme.

Q. *DR. JOHN I. INGLE*, Institute of Medicine: I'd like to ask Dr. Ahlberg how long it takes to train these particular assistants? Are they paid in comparison to a dental hygienist?

A. *DR. AHLBERG*: It didn't take long to train the women who were employed for the Lindhe-Axelsson investigation—a period of five to six weeks, if I remember correctly. Of course, they had previous formal training as dental assistants and had been practicing as such. But this only applies on an experimental basis. We haven't trained further numbers of such dental assistants; consequently, there have been no special negotiations regarding their salary level.

Q. *DR. LOIS COHEN*, National Institute of Dental Research: Dr. Ahlberg, do you have any information on enamel erosion which might be caused by frequent professional prophylaxis? My second question has to do with the Netherlands and the intriguing concept of their dental fitness card as a possible incentive for regular preventive visits to the dentist. Is there any information on the effectiveness of this plan?

A. *DR. AHLBERG*: With regard to enamel erosion, there exists no information indicating that erosion will occur due to professional cleaning. Moreover, I'd like to say that the tragic numbers of teeth lost to neglected periodontal disease are such that I would view very lightly the limited number of teeth that might be slightly damaged by enamel erosion due to excessive oral hygiene.

With regard to the dental fitness card in the Netherlands, I do not have any precise figures regarding its effectiveness. It is well supported by the profession, which feels this works very well, that patients are anxious to stick to their appointment service.

Q. *DR. EUGENE TRUONO*, practicing dentist, Wilmington, Delaware, and a member of the Council on Dental Care of the American Dental Association: Dr. Ahlberg, two questions, please. Is the Swedish dental insurance program a private insurance program or is it government insurance? Second, have you incorporated into that program a preventive mechanism that deals with plaque control as part of the concept?

A. *DR. AHLBERG:* The Swedish system is a government insurance system, although employers pay something like 85 percent of the cost. Yes, it's government assistance. In answer to your second question, yes, preventive plaque control as a principle is well included in the system.

Q. *DR. JOHN GREEN*, Chief Dental Officer, U.S. Public Health Service: Dr. Ahlberg, these are very impressive data you have presented. You talked about the prophylaxis in children and the effect on caries. As I interpret the data, you have also applied some fluoride to the children's teeth. Was there any attempt in the study to separate out the potential effect of plaque control versus making the teeth more resistant with fluoride?

A. *DR. AHLBERG:* Yes and no. You must remember that fluoride was applied in both test and control groups, but in different administrations. The control group received once a month supervised tooth brushing with an 0.2 percent sodium fluoride solution. The professional tooth cleaning occurred with a 5 percent monofluorophosphate abrasive paste every two weeks, so, of course, both the frequency and the amount of fluoride were greater there. However, it has not been possible to single out the effect of the fluoride. On the other hand, the difference in the results are so enormous that it's clearly not possible that fluoride was the main component in the success achieved on the test group. The objective of the study was not to single out one or more components of the preventive measures, but to study the effect of a whole appropriate oral hygiene program, including both professional tooth cleaning and, equally important, the home cleaning of the teeth.

Q. *DR. MELVIN RASKIN*, private dental practitioner, New York: Dr. Lennon, I understand that in England private health insurance is vital and growing. Can you tell us whether there is any private dental insurance and, if there is, can you draw any conclusions from its growth?

A. *DR. LENNON*: I can't really comment [on] how vital and growing medical insurance is; I don't know. Nor do we keep any detailed data on the private practice in dentistry. All I can say is that the gross income of dentists in the National Health Service seems to fall as the dentist to population ratio improves across the fifteen regions of England and Wales. It may be that those dentists in the better off dentist to population regions are doing private practice treatment. I don't know. The only private dental insurance I know about covers patients for nonpredictable dental catastrophies, like the need for gingivectomy or fractured jaw. Routine treatments are not included.

Q. *DR. JONATHAN NASH*, Thomas Evans Dental Institute, University of Pennsylvania: I presume that most of you from other countries know that the dental care situation in the United States is far from optimal. We are faced with maldistribution of dental personnel, and many people in the United States do not have proper access to dental care. Would any of you be bold enough to give us some suggestions that might improve matters here?

A. *DR. AHLBERG*: It is very difficult to reply to this question. In order to apply correctly the experience one can draw from other countries, one must be familiar with the country's social, cultural, and economical background, the manpower distribution, and so forth. One needs, in fact, to have proper epidemiological investigations before one can give a reply.

Q. *DR. GORDON WATSON*, executive director of the American Dental Association: First of all, I have found the meeting most stimulating and informative, and I want to compliment the planners of the session. I've enjoyed it a great deal. I've found, however, that in most of the areas from which we've had reports, very few of the countries parallel the problems, the size, the culture, or the financial status of our own country. And so for me, it has been difficult to make an overlay of our problems related to these reports. From my limited knowledge of West Germany, however, I have the impression that they most closely parallel some of our problems. They also have some innovative ways of financing their dental programs. I wonder if some thought had been given to a report from West Germany.

A. *DR. INGLE*:   Yes, Gordon, it was. As a matter of fact, Dr. Gillespie and I both tried to get someone here from West Germany, but the arrangement fell through at the last minute. We realize this was one of the deficiencies in our program, since Germany has the distinction of being a country where dentists are reported to earn more than physicians. We also wanted to have someone here from Israel, as well as East Germany, and the USSR. Although we had limited funds, we did make an attempt to get someone from West Germany.

Q. *DR. GILLESPIE*:   Dr. Kostlán, from your experience in working in the European region of WHO, have you any comments to make to Dr. Watson?

A. *DR. KOSTLÁN*:   Well, Mr. Chairman, I could comment very briefly with one reservation. I left the WHO service in 1973. So, if I may speak about the time preceding 1973, I would say that Western Germany might be considered the home country of private dental health insurance. It was in Germany where this insurance, if not invented, was applied for the first time. It has also spread the most, in terms of covering the population, getting the cooperation of the dental profession and expanding the scope of treatment. Dental health insurance started in Germany about 1890, spread moderately until 1920, and very fast afterward. Nowadays it has the cooperation of over 90 percent of the dentists. Purely private practice not covered by dental insurance is limited to about 5 percent in West Germany. German courts have even decided that fixed prosthetics should be covered by the dental health insurance. This is basically private insurance being financed fifty-fifty by insured persons and the employer. The families of the employees are included also, so practically the entire population is covered. I think the German dental profession is relatively happy with the insurance scheme.

Q. *DR. CHRISTINA KOCH*, American Dental Hygienists Association: I would like to make a comment, first about the practice of dentistry in West Germany. I've just recently returned from living in West Germany for two years and had the opportunity to practice traditional dental hygiene at the University of Munich. In providing care to patients, I had the opportunity to make many observations, especially in relation to the utilization of auxiliaries. First of all, utilization of auxiliaries is very limited in West Germany, although they are making attempts and efforts at this time to prepare auxiliaries to provide functions in traditional dental hygiene. At the present time, the German chairside dental assistant must undertake an additional six month training course to provide dental hygiene services to patients. Second, I have a couple of questions for Dr. Lennon. I am hoping he could provide some perspective on the utilization of auxiliaries in the national health service system, and second, if he will describe the New Cross dental nurse.

A. *DR. LENNON:* There are two forms of operating dental auxiliaries in the United Kingdom—the dental hygienist and the New Cross dental auxiliary. Their job descriptions are very clearly defined by regulation. The dental hygienist can work in the Hospital Service, the School Service, or in the General Dental Service. At present we have about 200—a handful. The New Cross dental auxiliary can only work in the School Dental Service, and she carries out simple restorative dentistry. The British Dental Association has recently stated their policy on dental ancillary workers, and they are of the opinion that dental hygienists should be trained in greater numbers, and that the New Cross scheme has not yet been fully evaluated and therefore should remain at the present level.

The government is taking active steps to increase the number of hygienists in training. We've had a recent report, The Court Report, into the whole of Child Health Services in England. The dental section of that report recommends that two new schools for New Cross dental auxiliaries should be built, but, to date, the government hasn't commented on that aspect of the report.

I might add that the arguments the BDA put against the New Cross auxiliary are really quite interesting. The arguments center on economics. As I explained in Chapter 12, we are already providing treatment in the United Kingdom cheaply. So, the BDA's first point is that the dentist is already efficient. The BDA believes that the differential between the cost of employing an auxiliary and employing another dentist is not as dramatic as it might at first appear. Second, one tends to compare the salary levels of the auxiliaries and the dentists, but to forget about operating expenses. A dentist with a net income of, say, £5,000 would also have operating expenses of £5,000, which would be the same for the dental auxiliary. Third, the BDA points out that recent legislation, the Equal Pay Act, requires that women should be paid the same wage for the same job as men. As a result, women's salaries in general are increasing. This will have an impact on the salaries of dental auxiliaries. In the future, says the BDA, dental auxiliaries will be able to command a salary at a commensurate level, so the differential may get even closer. The BDA's fourth argument relates to recruitment. If you are paying a dental auxiliary a rather low salary, there may not be a great incentive for her to come back to work after she's had a family. These arguments should be answered in the United Kingdom. I think, however, that the BDA's reason for putting them forward may not be entirely one of economics.

Q. *DR. JOHN HEIN*, Forsyth Dental Center: Dr. Ahlberg, the data you revealed of Jan Lindhe's work certainly makes for a fine review. This study is going to have a tremendous impact, and we ought to begin planning for it.

In view of the experiments going on with expanded function auxiliaries, it appears that Sweden is going to have a lot of human tragedy from having trained all those dentists. Are you beginning to think how Sweden must adjust to the impact of those preventive measures and titrate your manpower? Is this part of the plan?

A. *DR. AHLBERG*: That is right. I am no longer involved directly in Sweden, of course, but I know what is going on. Before I left Sweden in 1975, we asked the government to set up a study on the future distribution of dental manpower—that is, on the different types of auxiliaries in the dental team. This study is now under way. It's too early to say something about the results, but I think it's unanimous between the profession and the authorities in Sweden that we should employ more auxiliaries, particularly in the field of oral disease prevention.

Q. *DR. INGLE*: I'd like to ask myself a question that was asked of me during one of the coffee breaks. I showed that the primary teeth of the Chinese school children were in a terrible state of decay. The same fact was reported by Reginald Louie. When I got to the fourteen year olds, however, however, I found they have beautiful teeth—virtually no caries at all. The coffee break comment was, "Maybe the Chinese are doing this on purpose, just letting the deciduous teeth go, and the result is a fine set of caries-free permanent teeth." I've had other people tell me that this caries discrepancy is seen all over the Orient. My question is, What causes this phenomenon we are seeing? Does anyone have the answer?

A. *DR. LOGAN*: The breakdown of deciduous teeth is very, very common in the Pacific, the Polynesias, and in Southeast Asia. The thought is that it's probably due to a nutritional problem in early childhood.

Q. *DR. ALLEN HINDIN*: I'm not sure I can accept the idea that we are different from other countries. I think some of the children we see in our inner cities have just as many needs and perhaps just as great a problem as the children seen in South America or other parts of the world. Some of the adults in our rural areas probably experience the same problems as people in the outback. Dr. Ingle, is it your perception that we are indeed as different as we like to think we are?

A. *DR. INGLE*: I used a quote recently, and I wish I had it before me, because it says that there is something different about the United States. As I recall, it stated that New Zealand had social security forty-five years before it was passed in the United States. Germany had health insurance seventy-five years before it was even considered in the United States. England had gun control laws a hundred years before the United States even decided to talk about it. This article went down through a list of social programs that the United States either doesn't have or was very late in establishing in comparison to other countries of the world.

I'd have to say that what we've been talking about at this meeting is another manifestation of the lateness on the part of the United States to get into a social program that has been established in other parts of the world for generations. Dr. Kostlán pointed out that dental insurance programs started in Germany in the 1800s, and we didn't develop a dental service corporation in this country until 1954. By the same token, why are we so much different from our close neighbor, Canada, which probably holds the greatest similarity to the United States of any nation of the world? In the health care field, we are quite a bit different from Canada, and yet we think of ourselves as a very socially oriented nation, that we have an advanced social security system. Well, we might have, but it was very late in coming.

DR. LAWRENCE KERR, oral surgeon, Trustee of the ADA, Endicott, New York: I wonder if I might comment with some cobblestone philosophy. This nation was founded upon the basic tenet of total individual responsibility. Regardless of where our ancestors came from, the fact remains that they were all different. Some of those differences are changing; therefore, some of our philosophies will change. You've touched it exactly, we're all different, from politics to religion, to social, economic, and cultural differences. It was only in the late 1930s that we began any social welfare thinking. So, we're really a young nation just now beginning to suffer sociological problems, perhaps problems that other countries have experienced for a couple of thousand years.

Second, we would have to change our total incentive system, and we are an incentive-oriented nation, a nation economically oriented to a so-called free enterprise system that says, for what you do, you get. And if you don't do it so well, you don't get. Now we have a problem with forty million people who have not been getting regardless of what they do. There are those of us who will have a say in what the future shall hold in an ultimate health care delivery system. There is no way that the technology of dentistry alone will ever solve all these problems. I think that's the big lesson I'm going to take home.

Appendix

Participants at the Colloquium on International Dental Care Delivery Systems held in the National Academy of Sciences auditorium May 5 and 6, 1977, and sponsored by the Institute of Medicine and the Pan American Health Organization.

Program Speakers

Dr. Jan E. Ahlberg
Dr. Per Baerum
Dr. Gustavo Baz Diaz Lombardo
Dr. Lois K. Cohen
Dr. José Luis García-Gutiérrez
Dr. George M. Gillespie
Dr. David A. Hamburg
Dr. Harold Hillenbrand

Dr. John I. Ingle
Dr. Jarmil Kostlán
Mr. Michael Lennon
Dr. Michael H. Lewis
Dr. Richard K. Logan
Dr. Silvino Ruiz Miyares
Dr. Julius B. Richmond
Dr. Max H. Schoen

Program Moderators

Mr. Robert M. Ball
Dr. Chester W. Douglass
Dr. I. Lawrence Kerr
Dr. Alvin L. Morris
Mrs. Anne Scitovsky
Dr. Jeanne C. Sinkford

Participants

Dr. Howard L. Bailit
School of Dental Medicine
University of Connecticut
Farmington, Connecticut 06032

Dr. Ben D. Barker
Program Director
W.K. Kellogg Foundation
400 North Avenue
Battle Creek, Michigan 49016

Dr. Daniel Blandford
9312 Montpelier Drive
Laurel, Maryland 20811

Ms. Joyce E. Barnes
2615 Fairview Drive
Alexandria, Virginia 22306

LCDR A.E. Brandt DC USN
Section of Preventive Dentistry
NNDC—Washington Navy Yard
Washington, D.C. 20374

Dr. Jack Brown
11818 Charles Road
Wheaton, Maryland 20906

Dr. Ronald P. Burakoff
Room 3300—26 Federal Plaza
New York, New York 10028

Dr. N.R. Calhoun
1413 Leegate Road, N.W.
Washington, D.C. 20012

Dr. Louis Calisti
Harvard School of Medicine
188 Longwood Avenue
Boston, Massachusetts 02115

Ms. Isabella J. Chaplick, C.D.A.
RD 2, Box 312A, Heritage Road
Sewall, New Jersey 08080

Mr. Hal Christensen
Director, Washington Office
American Dental Association
1101 17th Street, N.W. (#10004)
Washington, D.C. 20036

Dr. Andrew Christopher
Chairman, Community Dentistry
Georgetown University
School of Dentistry
Washington, D.C. 20007

Mr. Norman Lee Clark
529 Clear Spring Road
Great Falls, Virginia 22066

Dr. Leonard Cohen
UMC School of Dentistry
2500 North State Street
Jackson, Mississippi 39218

Dr. Everod Coleman
Thomas Evans Dental Institute
University of Pennsylvania
Philadelphia, Pennsylvania 19104

Mr. Bernard J. Conway
Assistant Executive Director
  for Legislation
American Dental Association
211 East Chicago Avenue
Chicago, Illinois 60611

Dr. Neal A. Demby
RD #1
Worcester, New York 12197

Dr. Josue E. Diaz
Chief, Health Manpower Branch
U.S.P.H.S.—Region #2
Department of HEW
26 Federal Plaza—Room 3300
New York, New York 10003

Ms. Ann Dinius
Division of Dental Hygiene
School of Dentistry
Virginia Commonwealth University
MCV Health Sciences Center
Richmond, Virginia 23298

Rear Admiral Robert Elliott
Code 6, Dental Division
Bureau of Medicine and Surgery
U.S. Department of the Navy
Washington, D.C. 20372

Dr. Lewis Fox
1901 Residential
West Palm Beach, Florida 53401

Dr. William T. Fridinger
Allegany Community College
Cumberland, Maryland 21502

Dr. Sanford A. Glazer
8712 Victory Lane
Potomac, Maryland 20854

Dr. John C. Greene
Chief Dental Officer
U.S. Public Health Service
5600 Fishers Lane—Room 17–19
Rockville, Maryland 20857

Mr. M. Gudarzi
5620 Little Falls Road
Arlington, Virginia 22207

Dr. Joseph H. Hagan
Trustee, ADA District #6
Post Office Box #26
Crystal City, Missouri 63019

Dr. Ernest Hardaway, II
4620 North Park Avenue
Washington, D.C. 20015

Dr. John W. Hein
Post Office Box #156
Medfield, Massachusetts 02052

Dr. Lawrance D. Held
1032 West 38 SL
Erie, Pennsylvania 16508

Dr. Allen Hindin
19 Woodside Avenue
Danbury, Connecticut 06810

Dr. James R. Jensen
University of Minnesota
School of Dentistry
515 Delaware Street, S.E.
Minneapolis, Minnesota 55455

Ms. Brenda Johnson
Division of Health Ecology
School of Dentistry
The University of Minnesota
Minneapolis, Minnesota

Ms. Sara Johnson-Pena
909 Wootton Road
Bryn Mawr, Pennsylvania 19010

Dr. Anthony Jong
100 East Newton Street (7th floor)
Boston, Massachusetts 02118

Dr. Lireka Joseph
Department of Oral Health Care
   Delivery
School of Dentistry
University of Maryland
666 West Baltimore Street
Baltimore, Maryland 21201

Dr. Saul Kamen
Long Island Jewish-Hillside Medical
   Center
New Hyde Park, New York 11040

Dr. Dushanka V. Kleinman
6107 Melvern Drive
Bethesda, Maryland 20034

Ms. Christina M. Koch
American Dental Hygienist
  Association
Division of Dentistry
Federal Building #2
3700 East West Highway
Hyattsville, Maryland 20782

Dr. Isaac Konigsberg
University of Texas Health Science
  Center
Houston Dental Branch
Post Office Box #20068
Houston, Texas 77025

Mrs. Rosemary Lawnsby
444 Bedford Street
Stanford, Connecticut 06902

Dr. Robin M. Lawrence
U.S. Public Health Service
Region #1, Federal Building
Boston, Massachusetts 02203

Dr. A. John Lee
Regional Dental Director
Office of Regional Dental
  Consultant
1143 Sutherland Road
Kelowna, British Columbia

Dr. Elka S. Levin
6 Celadon Road
Owings Mills, Maryland 21117

Mrs. Jean Lewis
Lake George Road
RFD #3
Newton, Connecticut 06902

Ms. Judy Lewis
University of Connecticut
Department of Pediatrics
Farmington, Connecticut 06032

Ms. Martha Liggett
Department of Community Dentistry
Georgetown University
School of Dentistry
Washington, D.C. 20007

Dr. Roy L. Lindahl
305 Clayton Road
Post Office Box 2202
Chapel Hill, North Carolina 27514

Mr. Alfred Lindeman
Federal Trade Commission
Box 36005
450 Golden Gate Avenue
San Francisco, California 94102

Dr. Milton Linsansky
Acting Chief
Department of Dentistry
Yale-New Haven Hospital
789 Howard Avenue
New Haven, Connecticut 06504

Dr. Joseph Lipscomb
Duke University
Institute of Policy Sciences
4875 Duke Station
Durham, North Carolina 27706

Dr. Preston A. Littleton, Jr.
Division of Dentistry
Federal Center Building, #2
3700 East-West Highway
Hyattsville, Maryland 20782

Dr. Ralph R. Lobene
140 The Fenway
Boston, Massachusetts 02115

Dr. William C. Love
DCS Bureau of Community
  Health Services, HSA
Department of HEW
R7-30, Parklawn Building
Rockville, Maryland 20857

Dr. Jean-Paul Lussier
Dean, Faculty of Dental Medicine
Universite de Montreal
Box Office 6209, Succ. A.
Montreal, Quebec, Canada

Mr. John McCracken
Division of Dentistry
Health Resources Administration
3700 East West Highway
Hyattsville, Maryland 20782

Dr. Edwin E. McDonald
Bureau of Medicine and Surgery
Washington, D.C. 20372

Dr. Ralph E. McDonald
1121 West Michigan Street
Indiannapolis, Indiana 46202

Ms. Margaret B. McKinley
423 Warren Cres.
Norfolk, Virginia 23507

Dr. Henry L. Maines
10401 Old Georgetown Road
Bethesda, Maryland 20014

Dr. Robert Mecklenburg
10316 Gainsborough Road
Potomac, Maryland 20854

Dr. Rudolph Micik
Division of Dentistry
Federal Center Building #2
Room 3—22
3700 East West Highway
Hyattsville, Maryland 20782

Dr. and Mrs. William Milner
Route #3—Box 70
Pittsboro, North Carolina 27312

Dr. Jonathan Nash
The Thomas W. Evans Dental
  Institute
University of Pennsylvania
4001 Spruce Street A1
Philadelphia, Pennsylvania 19104

Mr. Kent Nash
Post Office Box 12194
Research Triangle Park
North Carolina 27709

Dr. Patricia Niles
Howard University
School of Dentistry
600 W Street, N.W.
Washington, D.C. 20059

Dr. W. Philip Phair
University of Iowa
College of Dentistry
Iowa City Iowa 52242

Ms. Hedy Quam
University of Minnesota
Program in Dental Hygiene
Minneapolis, Minnesota 55455

Dr. Melvin N. Raskin
3 Park Avenue
New York, New York 10016

Ms. Lindsay L. Rettie
652 Rosaer Lane
Virginia Beach, Virginia 23462

Dr. F.R. Rezai
5620 Little Falls Road
Arlington, Virginia 22207

Dr. Arthur L. Rudd
North 5901 Lidgerwood
Spokane, Washington 99207

Dr. Sheldon Rovin
Office of the Vice President
  for Health Affairs
The University of Washington
SC—61
Seattle, Washington 98195

Richard G. Rozier
Department of Health Administration
University of North Carolina
263 Rosenau 201H
Chapel Hill, North Carolina 27514

Capt. Henry J. Sazima, DC USN
OASD (Health Affairs) Pentagon
Washington, D.C. 20301

Cathy Schoen
Brookings Institution
1776 Massachusetts Avenue, N.W.
Washington, D.C. 20036

Dr. Hyman Schonfeld
1116 Caddington Avenue
Silver Spring, Maryland 20901

Dr. Selvin Sonken
Post Office Box 30172
Bethesda, Maryland 20014

Ms. Stanlee Joyce Stahl
Department of HEW
26 Federal Plaza
New York, New York 10007

Dr. Ward R. Stoops
14 Grove Street
Peterborough, New Hampshire 03458

Dr. Pasquale Tigani
916 19th Street, N.W.
Washington, D.C. 20006

Dr. Michael J. Till
School of Dentistry
University of Minnesota
515 Delaware Street, S.E.
Minneapolis, Minnesota 55455

Captain H.D. Tow, Jr., DC USN
Dental Division, Code 61—2
Bureau of Medicine and Surgery
Navy Department
Washington, D.C. 20372

Dr. Eugene J. Truono
Council on Dental Care Programs
American Dental Association
2300 Pennsylvania Avenue
Wilmington, Delaware 19806

Dr. R.D. Ulrey
Bureau of Medicine
U.S. Department of Navy
Washington, D.C.

Dr. Janet Urice
Maurice W. Perreault and Associates
1321 Connecticut Avenue, N.W.
Washington, D.C. 20036

Dr. H. Barry Waldman
School of Dental Medicine
Health Sciences Center
University of Stony Brook
Stony Brook, New York 11794

Dr. Robert R. Waller
Dental Section
Department of HEW
300 S. Wacker Drive
Chicago, Illinois 60606

Dr. Gordon C. Watson
Executive Director
American Dental Association
211 East Chicago Avenue
Chicago, Illinois 60611

Beatrice Weck
Department of Dental Hygiene
S.U.N.Y. at Farmingdale
Farmingdale, New York 11791

Dr. Harvey Webb, Jr.
President
National Dental Association
11108 Swansfield Road
Columbia, Maryland 21044

Dr. Martin Wohl
524 11th Street, S.E.
Washington, D.C. 20003

Ms. Rose P. Wooden
Academy of General Denistry
1050 17th Street, N.W.
Washington, D.C. 20036

Dr. Raymond F. Zambito
Chairman
Department of Dentistry
The Catholic Medical Center of
   Brooklyn and Queens, Inc.
88—25 153rd. Street
Jamaica, New York 11432

Index

About the Authors

John I. Ingle is a graduate of Northwestern University Dental School, with further specialty training at the University of Michigan. The author of a leading dental text, Dr. Ingle spent twenty-four years in academic dentistry; sixteen years at the University of Washington and eight years as dean of the School of Dentistry at the University of Southern California.

Dr. Ingle presently serves as Senior Professional Associate at the Institute of Medicine. As a worldwide consultant, his interest in international dental care delivery methods is broad and long standing.

Patricia Blair, who holds degrees from Wellesley and Haverford colleges, has written numerous articles and monographs on the economic, social and political development of the Third World. Her most recent project involved work with the National Academy of Sciences on preparations for the United Nations Conference on Science and Technology for Development. Formerly editor of Development Digest, Ms. Blair is a member of the international Governing Council of the Society for International Development.